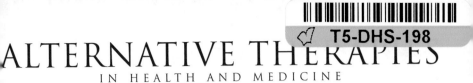

ALTERNATIVE THERAPIES
IN HEALTH AND MEDICINE

THE GONZALEZ PROTOCOL

Published by:
InnoVision Professional Media
3140 Neil Armstrong Blvd Suite 307
Eagan, MN 55121
E-mail: info@innovisionhm.com
www.innovisionhm.com

Publishers' note:
The information herein can be a valuable addition to your doctor's advice, but it
is not intended to replace the services of a trained professional. It is not safe to
self-diagnose. If you have symptoms suggestive of a condition discussed in this
book, please consult a health care practitioner.

Before experimenting with natural treatments, discuss them with your care
provider. Since many conventional health care practitioners may not be aware of
the natural alternatives available, you may need to help educate him or her. Bring
this book along with you to the doctor's office.

TABLE OF CONTENTS

Introduction

Colin A. Ross, MD

Several years ago, a friend of mine suggested that I read *The Trophoblast and the Origins of Cancer.*[1] He handed me his copy, and I opened it to the introduction. I was struck immediately by how much sense the trophoblast model of cancer makes: Here was a highly specified model of cancer formation rooted in research and with remarkable patient outcomes. I then recalled that I had read about Dr Gonzalez in Suzanne Somers's book, *Knockout.*[2]

Subsequently, I read Dr Gonzalez's other books and papers[3-5] and wrote 2 papers about his work.[6,7] I had lunch with him in New York in March 2015, at which time we discussed my 2 papers, which he and Dr Isaacs had read prior to my submitting them to journals. During the lunch conversation, Dr Gonzalez made an almost off-hand comment that illustrated the nature of his thinking about cancer. He said that chemotherapy selects for the most malignant cancer cells: Initially, the least malignant cells are killed off by the chemotherapy and there is a treatment response but, then, after a few months, the selected-for, more malignant cells that survived the chemotherapy take over, and the person declines rapidly and dies.

What an interesting and potentially important hypothesis! It may or may not be true, in many or some cancers, but it is a scientifically testable hypothesis, one that could be investigated in tissue culture, animal models, and humans. The idea is plausible, and there is a precedent for it with antibiotics and antibiotic-resistant bacteria, even though the mechanisms of antibiotic resistance must be very different from those in the response of cancer to chemotherapy. If Dr Gonzalez's idea is correct, in a subset of cancers, this by itself would be an important contribution to medicine, one that could affect both research and clinical practice.

As I read Dr Gonzalez's books, I also read the paper on the National Cancer Institute (NCI)-funded trial of pancreatic enzymes for treatment of pancreatic cancer[8] and visited the page about Dr Gonzalez on the NCI Web site.[i] The NCI Web site contains inaccurate and distorted information about the Gonzalez protocol. When I wrote to the NCI about these inaccuracies, it declined to make any revisions.

Also, I submitted my paper about the Chabot et al[8] trial to the journal that published it, *The Journal of Clinical Oncology*, and to the *Journal of the National*

---

i.   Please visit http://www.cancer.gov/about-cancer/treatment/cam/hp/gonzalez-pdq

Cancer Institute, both of which rejected it. I began to grasp the resistance Dr Gonzalez encountered from organized medicine throughout his career. The Chabot trial was plagued with so many problems—none of them acknowledged in the published paper, on which neither Dr Gonzalez nor Dr Isaacs were coauthors—that it should never have been published and should be disregarded. It purports to show that the treatment of pancreatic cancer with pancreatic enzymes is ineffective compared with chemotherapy. Problems include the fact that only 1 patient of 39 assigned to the pancreatic enzyme arm of the study fully complied with the protocol: 30 patients either took no enzymes, or followed the protocol incompletely or for a very short period. There were numerous such problems with the study.

The following is a typical outcome from Dr Gonzalez's practice:

> In January 1992, Ms S. found a mass in her abdomen and consulted her gynecologist. A CT scan showed a large pelvic mass, as well as 2 subcentimeter lesions in the hepatic dome. In February 1992, she underwent a total abdominal hysterectomy and bilateral oophorectomy. The pathology report showed a moderately differentiated serous cystadenocarcinoma; the tumor measured $10 \times 8 \times 4$ cm. She was advised to immediately begin aggressive chemotherapy because of the size of the tumor and the possibility of liver metastases. Her oncologist warned her that without chemotherapy, the cancer would prove deadly. Instead, she proceeded with Dr Gonzalez's treatment. An ultrasound of the abdomen and pelvis in August 1996 was completely clear, with no evidence of recurrent disease, or the previously described liver lesions. A CT scan of the abdomen and pelvis on June 29, 2009, done to evaluate her for kidney stones, describes the liver to be normal, without mention of the 2 hepatic lesions noted in the preoperative scan from January 1992, 17.5 years earlier.

At the time of his sudden death on July 21, 2015, Dr Gonzalez had completed a review of 106 such cases in an intended series of 150. It is, on the one hand, astounding that organized medicine ignores and discredits such results, and, on the other hand, business as usual. I doubt that there is a conventional oncologist anywhere who has these kinds of outcomes, in biopsy and MRI-confirmed advanced cases of highly malignant cancers. I imagine that one could survey a considerable number of oncologists, and all together they would have fewer survivors of stage III and IV pancreatic cancer alive after 10 years than Dr Gonzalez had in his practice. These outcomes cannot be accounted for by selection bias, spontaneous remission, or any other mechanism besides a treatment effect.

Week after week, we see reports in the media of celebrities who have been diagnosed with cancer. These are people with the supports and resources to be treated with the Gonzalez regimen. Most of them die. This is unnecessary. Many of these people (but not all) would be alive today if they participated fully in the

Gonzalez protocol. There is no rational, biological, medical, or scientific reason to ignore the treatment outcomes in Dr Gonzalez's practice. They are unmatched by any combination of surgery, radiation, and chemotherapy. Not only that, treatment responders, of whom there are many, start feeling better quickly on the Gonzalez regimen, which is very different from the quality of life experienced with surgery, radiation, and chemotherapy.

Is the Gonzalez regimen a panacea? No. Does it cure everyone? No. But it should be studied on a large scale, at the level of tens of millions of dollars. This is a gift to humanity that should not die with Dr Gonzalez. Dr Isaacs carries on alone, but she cannot practice forever. Given the resistance by organized medicine and oncology, most likely a private philanthropist is going to have to step forward.

I am very glad that my 2 papers were published before Dr Gonzalez died, so that he could read them, and I am very glad that I got to meet him in person. I have studied Dr Gonzalez's work because, like everyone, I have family members and friends who have died of cancer. I consider it my ethical obligation as a physician to speak up about the trophoblast model of cancer and Dr Gonzalez's work. Hence this special book by the publishers of *Alternative Therapies in Health and Medicine* in tribute to him. The special issue has relied on support provided by Andrew Campbell, MD; Mary Beth Gonzalez; Linda Isaacs, MD; and Kelly Brogan, MD.

The paper by Dr Gonzalez on a case of insulin-dependent diabetes, included in this book, was written by Dr Gonzalez prior to his death. Dr Gonzalez had been corresponding about his paper with Dr Campbell, the editor of *Alternative Therapies in Health and Medicine*, prior to his death. Dr Ross and Dr Brogan reformatted the paper for publication and did some light editing of it after Dr Gonzalez's death.

REFERENCES

1. Gonzalez NJ, Isaacs LL. *The Trophoblast and the Origins of Cancer: One Solution to the Medical Enigma of Our Time.* New York, NY: New Spring Press; 2009.
2. Somers S. *Knockout: Interviews with Doctors Who Are Curing Cancer—And How to Prevent Getting It in the First Place.* New York, NY: Three Rivers Press; 2010.
3. Gonzalez NJ. *One Man Alone: An Investigation of Nutrition, Cancer and William Donald Kelley.* New York, NY: New Spring Press; 2010.
4. Gonzalez NJ. *What Went Wrong? The Truth Behind the Clinical Trial of the Enzyme Treatment of Cancer.* New York, NY: New Spring Press; 2012.
5. Gonzalez NJ, Isaacs, LL. (1999). Evaluation of pancreatic enzyme proteolytic enzyme treatment of adenocarcinoma of the pancreas. *Nutr Cancer.* 1999;33(2);117-124.
6. Ross CA. The trophoblast model of cancer. *Nutr Cancer.* 2015;67(1);61-67.
7. Ross CA. Methodological flaws in the Chabot trial of pancreatic enzymes for the treatment of pancreatic cancer. *Int J Cancer Prev Res.* 2015;1;1-4.
8. Chabot JA, Tsai WY, Fine RL, et al. Pancreatic proteolytic enzyme therapy compared with gemcitabine-based chemotherapy for the treatment of pancreatic cancer. *J Clin Oncol.* 2010;28(12):2058-2063.

Dr Gonzalez as a Mentor: A Memoir

Kelly Brogan, MD

"Let the current system exist in a parallel universe and start from scratch with a completely new system that's based on nutrition, diet, psychology, and spirituality. We want a new medical model where prevention will be more important than treatment."

These are the words Nicholas Gonzalez, MD, after his untimely passing on July 21, 2015, has left thousands of patients, loved ones, followers, and colleagues breathless in despair. Here to shift the paradigm of health care as a teacher, author, and speaker, Dr Gonzalez devoted himself to this effort one patient at a time, every day, for 27 years of private practice. As one of the clinicians deeply and irrevocably transformed by knowing Dr Gonzalez, I will share my perspective on his journey and the gifts that he has left for us.

Nicholas Gonzalez, a proud American, born and raised in Queens by his Mexican father and Italian mother, graduated Phi Beta Kappa and magna cum laude, from Brown University in 1970, where he majored in English literature. Never interested in science, it wasn't until he began working as an investigative journalist assigned to interview some of the pioneers in nutritional and alternative medicine that he began to be inspired by geniuses such as 2-time noble laureate Linus Pauling, PhD. He decided to pursue medicine, turned down a book deal, and went to Cornell so that he could work with the then president of Memorial Sloan Kettering, Robert Good, MD, PhD, a transplant pioneer with an expressed interest in nutrition. It was under Dr Good's wing that Gonzalez was able to pursue the work of William Donald Kelley, dentist and clinical genius, much maligned in his own time and today. Gonzalez lived in his house and told me about being woken up at 4:00 in the morning to discuss science with this most unusual specimen of humanity. Dr Kelley treated and saved thousands of lives before he closed his practice, potentially withering into obscurity.

Dr Gonzalez's 5 years of research into Kelley's cases allowed for a better understanding of the optimal manufacturing of pancreatic enzymes for their anticancer effect. He describes this journey in his article, "The History of the Enzyme Treatment of Cancer,"[1,2] complete with 2 poignantly moving cases of successful long-term treatment of stage IV lung cancer and Burkitt's lymphoma. He greatly admired the work of John Beard, DSc (and was known to give 3-hour lectures on the subject) who first claimed that pancreatic enzymes (trypsin) have anticancer activity based on the trophoblast theory of cancer.[3] This theory has been supported by others such as Max Wicha, MD,[4] whose work has indicated that cancer does not arise from rogue mature cells, but from stem cells that lose regulatory control in a hostile, toxic environment.

After completing a fellowship in immunology, Dr Gonzalez started out on his own in 1987, despite being asked to work with Bob Atkins, MD, the famed weight loss doctor. He continued to care for a number of Kelley's long-term survivors and he became a sought-after clinician only a month into his private practice.

Today, there are thousands of patients touched by the work of Dr Gonzalez and his associate, Linda Isaacs, MD, most of whom are long-term survivors of advanced cancer.

Quick-witted and frank, Gonzalez once said,

> There is really only one truth. Either cancer patients get better with my treatment or they do not. And, if they do, I could not care less whether it involved moon dust or microbes from Pluto. What matters is that many—not all, by any means—of my patients are alive when they should be dead. And what has that made me in the eyes of the traditional cancer establishment? Simple. I am Gonzalez, the quack, the fraud, the doctor who lies to cancer patients, steals their money, and kills them. If there was a signup sheet at NIH to run me down with a truck, people would stand in line for hours.

Often accused of selection bias skewing his unprecedented results, Gonzalez reframed the relevance of doctor-patient alchemy stating, "Patients have to do the treatment they believe in. Fear is an infectious disease. You can catch fear but you can't catch faith. That has to come from within."

Requiring dietary adherence, daily enemas and detox methods, as well as upwards of 150 capsules per day, his protocol would not have been a "cure" for a patient otherwise oriented toward a quick chemical fix. The consummate teacher, Dr Gonzalez worked to liberate patients, not just from their illnesses, but to find their life's purpose and to thrive.

Dr Gonzalez was an activist and a deep supporter of health freedom. He had amassed an important and deeply undermining knowledge of the flaws in conventional research designed to support the use of cancer diagnostics and associated chemical treatments. Always a seeker of independent evaluation of his results, acknowledgement and validation by the medical establishment, Gonzalez was disillusioned by the mishandling of the Chabot trial, the details of which are discussed in a vindication recently published by a colleague.[5]

He nearly completed a compendium of 150 cases, meticulously documented, of patients made well by his protocol—a protocol he always attributed to his mentor, calling himself an "able technician." The cases will be published and should, if they are to be properly acknowledged, change the course of modern medicine.

All alternative practitioners know that food matters. But we are subject to the latest guru, some poorly designed study, or the lens of our own personal experience. Dr Gonzalez's approach offers patients a personalization of diet for regulation of all interconnected bodily systems. He used a 3-tiered approach of a personalized diet, detox, and supplementation, the core of which was glandular extracts.

He said that, "Anyone who recommends one diet to everyone hasn't studied the work of the great geniuses before us."

Kelley elucidated 10 dietary types on a map and also personally and clinically tested hundreds of nutrients for their properties in stimulating the parasympathetic and sympathetic arms of the nervous system. We have, as people, evolved in different ecological niches, with different relationships to the environment. The late microbiologist, René Dubos, PhD, was also an intellectual hero of Dr Gonzalez's, who among many brilliant quotes, stated:

> Man himself has emerged from a line of descent that began with microbial life, a line common to all plant and animal species . . . [he] is dependent not only on other human beings and on the physical world but also on other creatures—animals, plants, microbes—that have evolved together with him. Man will ultimately destroy himself if he thoughtlessly eliminates the organisms that constitute essential links in the complex and delicate web of life of which he is a part.

In these different niches, our nervous systems adapted to survive. Our ancestors interacted with the available food, the climate, and the microbes, and their bodies met and yielded to these forces like stone erodes from the waves. Those who survived, in time, had to be designed to complement the environment. From the Inuit to the Amazonians, the alkaline versus acidic nature of available foods selectively stimulated the 2 arms of the autonomic nervous system to perfectly balance it for survival in a given ecosystem.

There are those who thrive on a low-meat, high-leafy green and citrus diet, and those who thrive on a high-fat, meat-3-times-a-day regimen. Temperament and bodily habits can tell us a lot about where a given patient fits in this spectrum. In his time, Kelley subjected his patients to a 3200-question intake to help identify their type, but Gonzalez used specialized testing in his practice that served to support his clinical assessments.

I spent 7 months being mentored by Dr Gonzalez, and I count it as the most formative window of intellectual growth in my life. To be in his presence, to hear him speak, was to tap into a wisdom that I can only attempt to transmit in my time as a clinician. Suffice it to say that his clinical outcomes are unmatched the world over—that his knowledge base spanned the esoteric arts, biochemistry, and conventional cancer practice; there has not been a clinician yet who is as able to synthesize this material with the level of meticulous study he brought to each and every patient's journey. He had the gift of inhabiting the role of the healer—of materializing a path to lasting wellness for his patients—while also being a true intellectual and a visionary.

My intensive apprenticeship under Dr Gonzalez has inspired me anew. Case by case, I imagined the legions of patients who walked out of his office with the glorious lightness, and abiding gratitude, of those who have cheated death. Now, these patients contact me on a daily basis to share their deep sorrow at the loss of such a beacon of hope. They also, many of them, have already learned from him what they need to know to continue to survive and thrive even decades past their prognoses, but they know they will miss his companionship. He seemingly had an answer to every question in that otherworldly brain of his—every question except how we are meant to go on without him.

I dare say that my entire life has taken on a new meaning since knowing this man.

For this moment, I am so deeply grateful to have stood in his light. To have heard the truth he channeled—it's a sound so sweet; I hope to continue to share it with the world.

He always told me, "Your only job is to continue to love the truth, every day."

REFERENCES

1. Gonzalez NJ. Enzyme therapy and alternative cancer. Retrieved from http://www.dr-gonzalez.com/history_of_treatment.htm. Accessed July 31, 2015.
2. Gonzalez NJ. The history of the enzyme treatment of cancer. *Altern Ther Health Med.* 2014;20(S2):30-44.
3. Ross CA. The trophoblast model of cancer. *Nutr Cancer.* 2015;67(1):61-67.
4. Luo M, Clouthier SG, Deol Y, Nagrath S, Azizi E, Wicha MS. Breast cancer stem cells: Current advances and clinical implications. *Methods Mol Biol.* 2015;1293:1-49.
5. Ross CA. Methodological flaws in the Chabot trial of pancreatic enzymes for cancer therapy. *Int J Cancer Prev Res.* 2015;1:1-4.

Reporting on Dr Gonzalez for a Quarter Century: A Memoir

Peter Barry Chowka

Nicholas J. Gonzalez, MD ("Nick" to his friends) was, in this author's opinion, the most impressive and accomplished clinical practitioner of nutritional cancer therapy during the past 2 decades. In the early 1970s, I began covering the nascent field of alternative medicine. It was my privilege to meet, and to report on, many of the most notable innovative medical pioneers— including Linus Pauling, PhD; Mildred Nelson, RN; Dean Burk, PhD; and William Donald Kelley, DDS, who was destined to become Nick's mentor in nutritional therapies. After Nick began practicing medicine, he unquestionably became the peer of the best of these early pioneering clinicians and researchers.

During my first meeting with Nick in New York City in March 1990—an unforgettable encounter—it was immediately clear to me that he had the potential to do great work. He was smart, extremely dedicated, focused, energetic, without pretense—and very likable. For the next 2.5 decades, my first impressions of him never wavered.

With the support of his academic mentor, Robert A. Good, MD, PhD, the chief scientist, president, and director of the Sloan-Kettering Institute for Cancer Research in New York and widely credited as the founder of modern immunology,[1] Nick had spent 5 years evaluating and confirming the efficacy of Dr Kelley's enzyme-based, nutritional cancer therapy. In 1987, Nick and his partner, Linda Isaacs, MD, began practicing their version of Dr Kelley's therapy in Manhattan. It soon became known as the Gonzalez therapy. In early 1990, there was already a buzz about Nick in alternative medicine circles.

Prior to becoming a physician, Nick studied English and graduated with honors from Brown University. He worked as a journalist in New York and made his mark early on with a long investigative cover story in the July 31, 1972, issue of New York Magazine that exposed questionable goings on at an exclusive private prep school[2]; Nick's influential article led to the school's being closed down.

In 1978, Nick switched his career to medicine. Like many of the earlier, and most impressive, cancer therapy innovators, Nick embraced alternative medicine after first excelling in mainstream conventional academic medicine, which he found wanting, especially after he began investigating the work of Dr Kelley.

I had known and reported on Dr Kelley, dating from before the period when Dr Kelley gained national attention for treating actor Steve McQueen. McQueen had developed a deadly and conventionally untreatable form of lung cancer and there was evidence that Dr Kelley's therapy had helped him.[3] People who did not know Dr Kelley personally or who lacked an open mind might have easily dismissed the complicated and controversial clinician out of hand. In a field of iconoclasts, Dr Kelley was a quirky original and unconventional to the hilt. And yet, he impressed me and many others as a uniquely bright, compassionate, and caring man who had synthesized earlier innovators' work into a novel clinical model of treating cancer, and other diseases, exclusively with nutrition. In the 1970s and 1980s, Dr Kelley was widely known in alternative medicine circles as one of the most successful and outstanding innovative clinicians treating people with advanced cancer.

Nick respected Dr Kelley as much as I did—and this opinion that we shared helped to fast-track our lifelong friendship from the time when we first met.

During the 1990s, the first decade of our interaction, my conversations with Nick were mostly about the results of his (and Dr Isaacs's) promising results with cancer patients, which he always shared with great enthusiasm. Nick never failed to acknowledge and fully credit Dr Kelley's work as the basis for his own. I was less concerned with the details of the legal struggles that Nick was subjected to during the 1990s, because these sorts of distracting developments were par for the course: Almost every alternative clinician I had ever reported on, no matter how well motivated and credible (including Nobel Prize winners), had been targeted for hostile legal and government regulatory action on the part of opponents of clinical innovation.

In 1999 and for the next 5 years or so, the challenges of the 1990s gave way to a period that looked very promising for Nick. He seemed on the verge of mainstream recognition. His work found support among members of the US Congress.[4] The positive Gonzalez-Isaacs pilot study of pancreatic cancer patients was published in a scientific journal[5] and made national news, and the National Institutes of Health (NIH) had quickly followed suit with an unprecedented $1.4 million grant to fund a prospective clinical trial of the Gonzalez-Isaacs enzyme therapy under the direction of Columbia University.[6] It appeared that a high-level, objective, mainstream evaluation of the therapy was finally in the offing.

There was even a change in some of the mainstream media reporting about Dr Gonzalez's work. Most notably, in February 2001, *The New Yorker* magazine published a largely positive, 9000-word article about Nick, "The Outlaw Doctor," featuring a 2-page studio photo of Nick and 11 of his successfully treated patients.[7]

Before 5 years of the new century had elapsed, however, the government-funded study degenerated into a political morass and it would never be completed. In fact, an unfairly negative journal article about the unfinished study would be published in 2009, without Nick's or Dr Isaacs's participation or review.[8,9] Meanwhile, national health care reform was looming on the horizon while alternative medicine—the kind practiced by Drs Gonzalez and Isaacs—was being supplanted by complementary or integrative medicine.

A brief history is necessary here. In the 1970s and 1980s, nontoxic alternative cancer therapies represented a vigorous area of independent scientific inquiry and enjoyed considerable popularity with the American public. Pockets of promising clinical innovation ranged from New England and New York City, across the continent to California and south of the border to Tijuana, Mexico, which, for a time, was known widely as a healing Mecca. In the early 1980s, Dr Kelley had a presence at an alternative cancer clinic in Baja California, Mexico. Alternative cancer's leading proponents and its most popular therapies were frequently in the news and hundreds of thousands of Americans supported the concept of medical freedom and for a time composed a viable grassroots political movement that was active on behalf of medical freedom of choice.[10]

Looking back, the period was a Renaissance of alternative medicine— especially alternative cancer—and it represented the high point for the field of primary alternative cancer treatments in the United States. The disfavor that the medical establishment and its allies—including government bureaucracies, academic medicine, and the pharmaceutical industry—have always heaped on the proponents of medical alternatives took new and different strategic turns starting around 1990.

On the heels of the US Government Office of Technology Assessment's flawed 1990 study *Unconventional Cancer Treatments*,[11] which gave Dr Kelley's and Dr Gonzalez's work short shrift, the US Congress, with good intent, created and funded at the NIH a brand new Office for the Study of Unconventional Medical Practices, later changed to the Office of Alternative Medicine (OAM). But instead of validating credible alternatives, which the Congress intended as the OAM's primary mission,[12] the OAM and the much larger agencies it morphed into ultimately served to diminish the availability of many primary clinical alternatives. The inexorable path downhill to this ignominious outcome was long and convoluted. The original, independent-minded pioneers were getting old and passing on, and the new generation of young proponents tended to be susceptible to seduction and co-optation by federal agencies proffering the lure of generous funding grants and—after decades of disregard—a smattering of official approval. A watering down, or winnowing, of the primary alternative therapy model was beginning to take hold.

In 1981, Albert Szent-Gyorgyi, MD, PhD, who was awarded a Nobel Prize in 1937 for his discovery of vitamin C, and who, in the last years of his life, was working on alternative cancer therapies but was getting little attention, cautioned me: "The purpose of science and medicine has become not to make discoveries but to get grants granted."[13] Szent-Gyorgyi was talking about conventional science and medicine. But within a decade, the proliferation of government grants that were suddenly being made available to alternative clinicians and researchers began to influence and permanently alter the landscape of alternative medicine, as well. Inspired by the government's new largesse, a variety of much more palatable—and fundable—models of complementary alternative medicine (CAM) and integrative medicine emerged. This new, nonthreatening alt med "light" started to replace primary alternative medicine, which was unfortunate because it was primary alternative medicine that had inspired the promising, paradigm-changing challenges to conventional medicine to begin with.

In a sign of the times, the OAM changed its name to the National Center for Complementary and Alternative Medicine and then to the National Center for Complementary and Integrative Health. In this newly evolving scientific and political milieu, Nicholas Gonzalez stuck to his principles and continued to practice his primary alternative (rather than complementary or integrative) treatment approach, but he was not always in sync with the times.

The record of Gonzalez's largely unsuccessful 2-decade quest for fair evaluation of his work is well documented, including in his 2012 book, *What Went Wrong*.[14] In particular, the collapse of the NIH's clinical trial of the Gonzalez-Isaacs therapy is merely one of the most recent examples of how government-funded tests have always treated promising medical alternatives going back decades (including Linus Pauling's work on vitamin C).[15] It's also emblematic of the systemic obstruction that continues to be placed in the path of primary alternative treatments to this day.

Notwithstanding the myriad and never ending obstacles and disappointments, during all of the years that I knew him, Nick remained upbeat and doggedly focused on his work—treating patients, seeking new clinical insights, keeping up with the state of the art in science and medicine, writing articles, responding to media requests, and lecturing. According to Nick, his status as "one man, alone" (the title of an article about him that I published in 2002, inspired by the title of Nick's own book about Dr Kelley) changed in 2001 when he met and married the talented, accomplished, and dedicated Mary Beth Pryor. With her support and assistance, Nick became even more prolific, and he wrote or coauthored 4 major books between 2009 and 2012. He was nearing completion of his latest work, presenting over 100 of his best cases, when he passed away suddenly on July 21, 2015.

In recent years, as the last of the original alternative cancer pioneers left the scene, Nick and I frequently commiserated privately about the fact that truly alternative, primary natural approaches to treating cancer were becoming harder and harder to find. This realization seemed to increase Nick's sense of urgency and dedication to documenting the details of his therapy and its clinical successes in order to leave a signpost for the future of medicine.

During the last decade, I often compared notes with Nick—and I published several long interviews with him—about larger issues affecting the future of medicine in society. We agreed that handing the direction and control of medicine over to large bureaucracies was a prescription for disaster that would adversely influence clinical innovation and the sanctity and success of the doctor-patient relationship. Still, Nick was convinced that in time (he often cited the implosion of the Soviet Union as evidence) the momentum toward socialized medicine would be seen for what it is—a Faustian bargain—and be replaced by the public's support for a return to a more traditional American model of competition, medical freedom, and personal responsibility.

Nick always maintained an optimistic public, and private, persona. In late 2014, in the course of 3 months, Nick and I exchanged more than 200 e-mails. He was working on his magnum opus—the collection of his best cases—and he was in a very reflective frame of mind. Our wide ranging discussions included issues and personalities in medicine and his motivation. He confirmed that the patients whom he and Dr Isaacs had successfully treated throughout the years kept him grounded and focused on his practice, no matter what the controversies of the moment. In addition, Nick cited his deep Christian faith that was further reinforced by his extensive knowledge of Biblical scholarship.

Nick wrote in an e-mail to me on September 25, 2014:

> You inquired how I could stand the criticism. It's only because of God, and my belief in Him. God led me to Kelley, and I trust Him completely. If He wants my work to survive, it will survive, no matter how stupidly I personally behave. If He doesn't want it to survive, it won't, no matter how perfectly and smart I behave. It's all up to Him. My job is to do the best job possible.

The death of a friend such as Nick Gonzalez was not only a disorienting shock on a personal level to everyone who knew him—it was deepened by the realization that the important work of this remarkable individual had come to an end. Considered in retrospect, several months later now, his extraordinary accomplishments are highlighted anew and brought into clearer focus. Nick's thoughts and words as I recorded and documented them, and as he shared them in his prolific writings and in other interviews and media appearances, all assume new and profound levels of meaning and importance.

In reality, Nicholas Gonzalez's work has not ended. Like all great men and women, his legacy survives him. A large part of that legacy and a testament to his success are the people who Nick helped or cured of cancer and who are alive to this day, long after their original prognoses predicted they would be dead. Fortunately, Nick was not only a remarkable clinician and a healer of the sick—he was an equally talented and inspired writer and speaker. The considerable body of work that he left us, including the many interviews, will, I expect, continue to inform, enlighten, and inspire both laypeople and a new generation of healers—

aided by the efforts of his widow, Mary Beth Gonzalez, committed to helping to keep the recognition of Nick's work alive and growing; and by his colleague and close friend of 30 years, Dr Linda Isaacs, who remains in clinical practice in New York, offering the continued promise of the Gonzalez-Isaacs therapy.

REFERENCES

1. Wright P. Robert Alan Good. *Lancet.* 2003;362(9390):1161.
2. Gonzalez NJ. Showdown at Sands Point. *New York Magazine.* July 31, 1972:36-43.
3. Chowka PB. Steve McQueen: Legacy of a medical outlaw. *New Age.* 1981;6(7):28-37.
4. No author listed. Burton Lauds Gonzalez's research results in fighting pancreatic cancer. http://tinyurl.com/burton-lauds-gonzalez. Published June 25, 1999. Accessed October 8, 2015.
5. Gonzalez NJ, Isaacs LL. Evaluation of pancreatic proteolytic enzyme treatment of adenocarcinoma of the pancreas, with nutrition and detoxification support. *Nutr Cancer* 1999;33(2):117-124.
6. Chowka PB. Government funds test of the Gonzalez nutritional cancer therapy. http://tinyurl.com/1999-gonzalez-test. Published August 15, 1999. Accessed October 8, 2015.
7. Specter M. The outlaw doctor. *The New Yorker.* February 5, 2001:48-61.
8. Chabot JA, Tsai WY, Fine RL, et al. Pancreatic proteolytic enzyme therapy compared with gemcitabine-based chemotherapy for the treatment of pancreatic cancer. *J Clin Oncol.* 2010;28(12):2058-2063.
9. Ross CA. Methodological flaws in the Chabot trial of pancreatic enzymes for cancer therapy. *Int J Cancer Prev Res.* 2015;1(1):1-4.
10. Petersen JC, Markle GE. Politics and science in the Laetrile controversy. *Soc Stud Sci.* 1979;9(2):139-166.
11. US Government Printing Office. *Unconventional Cancer Treatments.* US Congress, Office of Technology Assessment, OTA-H-405. Washington, DC: US Government Printing Office; September 1990.
12. Boyle EW. The politics of alternative medicine at the National Institutes of Health. Federal History Online. http://tinyurl.com/boyle-politics-am. Published 2011. Accessed October 8, 2015.
13. Chowka PB. Is alternative medicine dead? http://tinyurl.com/2005altmed-dead. Published March 1, 2005. Accessed October 8, 2015.
14. Gonzalez NJ. *What Went Wrong: The Truth Behind the Clinical Trial of the Enzyme Treatment of Cancer.* New York, NY: New Spring Press; 2012.
15. Richards E. The Politics of therapeutic evaluation: The vitamin C and cancer controversy. *Soc Stud Sci.*1988;18(4):653-701.

Dr Gonzalez as a Spouse: A Memoir

Mary Beth Gonzalez

Nick Gonzalez had a lot to say and, fortunately for us, he openly shared his opinions. I'll start this tribute to my dear husband with an excerpt written by Nick for our family's quarterly newsletter. Our April, 2015, theme was "Blessings" and here is Nick's submission:

> To me, the greatest blessing is, of course, life itself, the great gift God has given to us all. In the day to day happenstance of our lives, we take the fact of our life so often for granted, understandably, with the ebb and flow of each day's events. But I myself never take my life, or those I know and love for granted, I thank God for this blessing every day.
>
> Though I take full credit, and full responsibilities, for my conscious and free will mistakes, I give God credit for salvaging me repeatedly from the errors of my ways, and bestowing on me gifts and benefits and yes, blessings, I hardly deserve or have earned out of my own independent action and thought. God gave me my abilities, however expansive or limited they might be, he blessed me with an inquisitive mind, the capacity for determination to see difficult projects through to the end, the capability to overcome seemingly impenetrable and insurmountable obstacles that have come my way over the years. In a very practical sense, I have chosen, with God's guidance, a difficult career path for sure, taking on it seems at times the entire conventional medical world. Though I am a very small David in comparison to the Medical Pharmaceutical alliance, I and my treatment still survive, I still have many patients, told they were going to die, turn around and live and achieve excellent good health. It is indeed a great blessing, to witness these patients survive and succeed, over and over again, during the past 27 plus years of my medical practice. And with God's help and blessing, my work continues to grow in prominence, silencing or at least minimizing the complaints of the critics.
>
> I feel so blessed that Mary Beth came into my life, to bring a personal security and fulfillment previously lacking. Her belief in my work, her steadfastness beside me as I take on the world, means more than I can say, and is a blessing I never would have expected. Her deep Christian faith is also a blessing, cementing our marriage, our friendship, and our love, with the acknowledgement that God rules and oversees all, including our marriage.
>
> These blessings, and there are many more, have been given me freely, out of God's grace, through no effort or achievement on my part. They always come, it seems, always at the most important time in my life, when the gifts given fulfill an immediate need. I know such workings in my life are not the result of chance, but only the graciousness of God, his blessing, given me for whatever reason he chooses to do so.

All of you, no matter how difficult life might seem at the present, how frustrating the world now or the future may seem, should remember the gifts we do have, the blessings we have been allotted, these gifts from God, which should give us strength for today's tasks and battles, and for those we face tomorrow. For in my experience, when least expected, another blessing, perhaps small, perhaps large, will suddenly make itself evident in my life, bringing with it joy, and fulfillment, and always greater hope.

How blessed am I now to have his words of encouragement to a battle that he hadn't predicted and one for which he and I had no plan.

Throughout our marriage, Nick and I were a team. We cherished each other and supported our individual careers. However, I soon came to realize that despite the importance of my marketing career, my calling was to make Nick's life as easy as possible so that he could fulfill his destiny to help so many people.

As a very young man, Nick believed that he was given a gift and he had a special mission while on Earth. In his daily personal relationship with God, The Holy Spirit guided him. This guidance fueled Nick's work and gave him great strength, and it also enabled Nick to know something about literally everything. I was constantly astounded to hear Nick speak as intelligently about politics and Bach, global warming and Mickey Mantle's baseball's stats as he could about the latest from the Kardashians and Miley Cyrus. I used to laugh with him and ask whether he really was going to the office every day or perhaps he was simply sitting around reading *US Magazine*. He'd belly laugh at the thought and his eyes would dance and twinkle.

Nick knew that he was destined to write a very important book that would change the course of medicine. Nick had already published 3 books and was working most nights and weekends on a massive 3-volume book of 125 of his best patient case reports. He had completed 106 meticulously documented medical miracle cases of all types of cancer and other diseases. I repeatedly suggested that perhaps 100 cases would be sufficient, and we could start the publishing process. But Nick truly measured success in lengths of time and volume. So it will come as no surprise that a book of 100 patient cases was just not enough. Nick knew that 125 cases was the right number. Now, we will publish his case book to fulfill his destiny and for all humanity.

Nick lectured about his work all over the world. He loved to teach and share his knowledge to anyone who would listen. When lecturing, he was known to ignore his time limit and announce as he was being given the hook—the 2-minute warning: "I'll just keep on talking and I won't be upset if you have to leave." Nick often received thunderous standing ovations after his lectures with crowds of people following him back to his hotel room to thank him and ask questions.

What do we do now without him here to answer our questions? First, we need to question what we hear from conventional medicine. We need to listen to Nick's teachings through his books, lectures, and interviews. And as patients, we need to listen to our bodies. We need to continue to do our protocols and practice what we have been taught. Finally, we need to celebrate Nick's life and his pioneering contributions to the history of medicine.

Like many who knew him, I became aware within minutes of meeting Nick that he was uniquely gifted. I gladly—willingly—encouraged Nick to share his gifts with the world. Some people go their whole lives not finding love. I am blessed that every day for 14 years, I knew that Nick adored me. I know that he too felt blessed that we found each other, and now I live in that twinkle in his eye which will never, ever die.

I am comforted, and maybe you will be, too, by the words the Reverend Terence Elsberry spoke at Nick's funeral service.

> Nick spent his adult life walking in the spirit of Jesus to bring healing wherever he could. Healing was Jesus's passion. Healing was Nick's passion. Our faith tells us Nick is okay. He's more than okay. And he's alive. If we could see him, we'd see how vibrantly alive he is.
>
> And he's really not all that far from us. We can talk to him and know he hears us. We can see his presence in the most unexpected places and ways that remind us that he's always with us. Because God loves us. He loves Nick. And love is forever.
>
> There's something else. God gives us things to do in heaven. We are not just laid on a shelf to indulge in some kind of celestial slumber. Can you imagine Nick Gonzalez sleeping through eternity? He will not. The gifts and talents Nick had in this life he still has in the next.
>
> Which means to me that somehow, in some way that we'll understand not now but down the road, God is going to still be making use of Nick's brilliant mind and his passionate caring. Who's to say that heaven doesn't have healing agents who come to us in this life to heal us and inspire doctors and healers of all kinds with heavenly wisdom they would have in no other way? For me, there is no doubt: Nick is still sharing the blazing light of his knowledge and his power and his love from that realm to this. God reigns! Nick lives! The healing continues!

I know that Nick's work will someday be validated and recognized as the most direct way to finding wellness. God designed us to be well. Nick taught us how to achieve it. And I know that when Nick met God, he heard the words all of us hope to one day hear: "Well done, good and faithful servant" (Matthew 25:23, King James Version).

Dr Gonzalez as a Colleague: A Memoir

Julian Hyman, MD

In the late 1980s, I was contemplating my retirement from my medical practice when I received a call from Dr Jonah Goldstone, who served with me in the Department of Oncology at Roosevelt Hospital. He knew about my plans and asked whether I would like to take over on an interesting problem that he believed would be a good match for me.

Dr Goldstone had been hired as an expert for a case of a physician who was practicing serious alternative medicine and was told that his license to practice was being revoked by the Professional Medical Board on the basis of a complaint filed by another physician.

Dr Goldstone was then hired to represent Dr Nicholas Gonzalez in a court of law. At the hearing, it was decided that Dr Gonzalez would be given 1 year to prove that he deserved to maintain his practice of medicine. Part of this process was developing a program of study about treatments for patients with malignancies. This would have to be coordinated with a physician who was accepted by the New York State Board. After much thought, I realized this was a significant opportunity and was then accepted by the board to take on this role.

I was told that at any time during the duration of this program, Dr Gonzalez could be examined without notification and would be observed by a member of the State of New York Board of Medical Examiners and also by the Professional Board of New York State.

I agreed to these conditions and arranged to visit Dr Gonzalez at his office in Manhattan. We worked out a plan that was acceptable to both of us, and this included a weekly visit to his office at a time when a patient was there for a follow-up evaluation.

It was evident that he had excellent medical training. He was a graduate of Cornell Medical School. Following his graduation, he continued to study with an expert from the university who interested him in the importance of diet. This led to his interest in alternative medicine.

Part of our plan also included a weekly visit to the Oncology Clinic at Roosevelt Hospital. At first, Roosevelt did not want to accept hosting this program because Dr Gonzalez was not on the staff there, but I was able to negotiate with the head administrator and they became willing to make an exception that was a very important piece in this process. At the clinic sessions, we looked at many types of malignancies, although pancreatic cancer was the area of special interest for Dr Gonzalez.

The third part of our plan was to visit an oncologist who had shared an office with me. This enabled Dr Gonzalez to observe a more traditional approach to treatments. The visit to the clinic required a complete history and physical examination and a complete discussion of the case. One day, there was a surprise visit from 2 representatives of the State Board and the Professional Medical Board of New York. Dr Gonzalez did so well that they never believed they needed to examine him again. I kept up by sending frequent reports to the New York State Department of Medical Examiners.

Following the completion of the year, the Professional Board of Examiners dismissed the charges and reinstated Dr Gonzalez's medical license. After this meaningful outcome, there were still a few patients who were suing Dr Gonzalez for possible malpractice.

Because I believed in his work, I was willing to go to court as a professional witness. I was pleased to learn that many of these cases ended favorably. Although I trained and practiced only traditional approaches to treatment of malignant disease, I learned from Dr Gonzalez that the practice of alternative medicine could also be effective.

From the time I first met Dr Gonzalez, I was impressed by his level of integrity and caring. It was clear that he was always extremely devoted to the individual needs of his patients. The patients I met all seemed very confident in the care they received. It impressed me that the results of his treatment indicated that many of his patients were doing better than their predicted life expectancy.

We often had lunch together in a small kitchen in his office. We talked about his family and his interest in music and also in American history. His family came from Italy and they were particularly interested in classical music. For a short period, he played a classical instrument.

When all of these cases were resolved, Dr Gonzalez and I established a lasting friendship. We both respected each other and continued to see each other and included my wife and his wife, Mary Beth Gonzalez, at these very pleasant meetings. We continued to discuss medical problems that involved both of us.

His sudden passing is a huge loss to his family, friends, and patients. Fortunately, Dr Gonzalez had trained a colleague, Dr Linda Isaacs, who can continue with his protocols.

Dr Gonzalez as a Practice Colleague: A Memoir

Linda L. Isaacs, MD

As I was finishing my internal medicine training in 1991, the other residents in my year were discussing their future plans for fellowships in various subspecialties. But there was no doubt in my mind about my next step: I was going to work with Nick Gonzalez in his nutritional practice.

I had met Nick when I was a medical student and he was an intern at Vanderbilt University Medical Center. At that time, he was engaged in studying the work of William Donald Kelley, a brilliant and controversial dentist who had developed an alternative treatment protocol for cancer. Nick had told me about some of the cases he had discovered in Dr Kelley's files: a patient with widespread prostate cancer who had been admitted to the hospital for pain control, who after beginning the Kelley program had completely recovered; a patient with uterine cancer metastatic to the lungs whose disease had completely regressed after starting the treatment plan Dr Kelley had given her; and many more. As a medical student, I had been impressed, but by the time I had completed my internal medicine residency, I had a more solid understanding of how unusual these patient histories were, because I had seen the relentless downhill course of similar patients in my training.

By this time, Nick had been in practice in New York City for several years, working to recreate Dr Kelley's methods and collecting case histories of his own. I joined him in his small shared office space on Park Avenue; there was no space for me to see my own patients, but there was plenty to do. Every night, I would listen to him return telephone calls from patients, learning the management skills he had developed to help patients deal with the implementation of their nutritional protocols. And during the day, I reviewed the charts of successful patients, studying Nick's treatment plans, and working to collect any documentation the patients or their physicians had not previously provided.

The year 1993 was eventful for us. Nick was contacted in the spring, by the then associate director of the Cancer Therapy Evaluation Program at the National Cancer Institute (NCI), inviting him to present cases. With my assistance, Nick compiled 25 cases into a short monograph. This presentation included some very striking stories, such as a woman with breast cancer metastatic to the liver and brain, with documented resolution of disease on the therapy; and a man with renal cancer who had a metastatic lesion the size of an egg protruding from his skull, whose tumor regressed after he began his protocol.

In July, 1993 he traveled to Bethesda, Maryland, with a heavy bundle of supporting documents and films, to speak to a group of NCI scientists. After the session, the associate director suggested a pilot study with pancreatic cancer, though no funding for such a study was volunteered. Shortly thereafter, funding was provided through Dr Pierre Guesry at Nestlé, and the study began in September, 1993. At the same time, we were able to move into new office space that gave me room to see patients myself. Nick and I would work together there for the next 22 years.

The pilot study ended in 1998, and the results were published in the June 1999 issue of *Nutrition and Cancer*.[1] Of 11 patients followed in the trial, 8 of 11 suffered stage IV disease. Nine of 11 (81%) lived 1 year, 5 of 11 lived 2 years (45%), 4 of 11 lived 3 years (36%), and 2 lived longer than 4 years. In comparison, in a trial of the drug gemcitabine, of 126 patients with pancreatic cancer, not a single patient lived longer than 19 months.[2]

In 1998, the NCI, in conjunction with the National Center for Complementary and Alternative Medicine, approved funding for a large-scale, controlled trial evaluating our approach against chemotherapy, again in patients diagnosed with pancreatic cancer. Unfortunately, despite our initial enthusiasm for the project, it was ineptly managed by the academicians involved, who published an article about it without our consent in 2009.[3] Nick's book, *What Went Wrong: The Truth about the Clinical Trial of the Enzyme Treatment of Cancer*,[4] details the problems with the trial quite thoroughly, and it spells out why we did not think the published paper's results were valid.

This was a bitter disappointment for both of us, but we had seen too many miraculous results in our office to choose to give up. Nick's favorite word to describe himself was *relentless*, and he would live up to this in the following years. In the January/February 2007 issue of *Alternative Therapies in Health and Medicine*,[5] we published a series of 31 case histories of successfully treated patients. Nick also finally published his monograph about Dr Kelley's work[6] and a book on the science backing the use of pancreatic proteolytic enzymes for cancer.[7] At the time of his death, he was working on a lengthy book of patient cases.

In the days after his death, as I struggled in the midst of my own grief to care for those who already had appointments booked and plane reservations made, his patients expressed so much gratitude for his devoted care that had transformed their lives. Their stories help give me the determination to do what I can to keep Nick's memory alive and to continue the work so that perhaps a future generation of researchers can pick up where we left off.

REFERENCES

1. Gonzalez NJ, Isaacs LL. Evaluation of pancreatic proteolytic enzyme treatment of adenocarcinoma of the pancreas, with nutrition and detoxification support. *Nutr Cancer.* 1999;33(2):117-124.

2. Burris HA, Moore MJ, Andersen J, et al. Improvements in survival and clinical benefit with gemcitabine as first-line therapy for patients with advanced pancreas cancer: A randomized trial. *J Clin Oncol.* 1997;15(6):2403-2413.

3. Chabot JA, Tsai WY, Fine RL, et al. Pancreatic proteolytic enzyme therapy compared with gemcitabine-based chemotherapy for the treatment of pancreatic cancer. *J Clin Oncol.* 2010;28(12):2058-2063.

4. Gonzalez NJ. *What Went Wrong: The Truth Behind the Clinical Trial of the Enzyme Treatment of Cancer.* New York, NY: New Spring Press; 2012.

5. Gonzalez NJ, Isaacs LL. The Gonzalez therapy and cancer: A collection of case reports. *Alt Ther Health Med.* 2007;13(1):46-55.

6. Gonzalez NJ. *One Man Alone: An Investigation of Nutrition, Cancer, and William Donald Kelley.* New York, NY: New Spring Press; 2010.

7. Gonzalez NJ, Isaacs LL. *The Trophoblast and the Origins of Cancer: One Solution to the Medical Enigma of our Time.* New York, NY: New Spring Press; 2009.

A Tribute to Dr Nicholas Gonzalez

An Anonymous Patient

I first heard of Dr Nicholas Gonzalez on Feb 4, 1989, when I was lying in a hospital bed just diagnosed with ovarian cancer, stage IV. I was 1 day postsurgery, having been admitted with a large mass of unknown origin. My oncologist advised me to have the traditional treatment of chemotherapy and scheduled me to begin that weekend. I was not interested in having chemotherapy, being a registered nurse and knowing what effects it has on the immune system, so I was very upset. I knew I needed to fight this disease with all the strength I had and destroying my immune system was not the way! I didn't know what to do, but I was sure I wasn't going the route of chemo; my nurse friends suggested tamoxifen, because it was newly discovered and thought to be effective in fighting the disease.

Then into the hospital room walked one of my friends who had researched Dr Gonzalez because her father had pancreatic cancer and died before he could be scheduled. She brought me the book by Dr Kelley,[1] and I was very interested! Here, I thought, was my answer! I thought I would call and try the program, and, if it didn't work, I could always go "back to chemo."

From the very first meeting, Dr Gonzalez instilled confidence in me and gave me a feeling of hope and optimism. It all just made sense to me and I felt this was going to work from the beginning. I felt it was the answer to my prayers.

I knew it was going to be a lot of work, but I was not one to shirk from work. Most important, it was a "clean" treatment program, using the body's natural defenses and building the immune system, not destroying it. I was not introducing harmful chemicals into my body.

I began feeling better and better with each visit. Today, I am a strong, vital, healthy woman at 76 years of age. Dr Gonzalez was always available to me for questions, anytime, related to cancer or not. He provided advice to me or made a referral to another expert in the field. He always returned my calls and, most important, I knew he cared.

A genius with a probing mind and generosity of spirit, I believe I am alive today and my good health and lack of evidence of cancer in my life are due to him and his fortitude in carrying out the program despite lack of support from the medical complex.

REFERENCE

1. Kelley WD. *One Answer to Cancer*. Los Angeles, CA: Cancer Book House; 1969.

Testimony From a Grateful Family

An Anonymous Spouse

"Greater love has no one than this: to lay down one's life for one's friends."
(John 15:13, New International Version)

Isn't this what Nick Gonzalez did for his patients? We heard the Earth-shattering news about Nick's death just a few weeks ago. And ever since, I couldn't stop thinking about how Christ-like he was.

In the same way Jesus stood up to the religious leaders of his day, Nick stood up to the pharmaceutical and conventional medical industries of our day. His words were profound yet delivered in humility. He was a rebel, a healer, a miracle worker, a teacher, a truth-teller. And to so many, including my husband and me, a hope-giving savior.

On September 28, 1988, the day before our daughter was born, my husband was diagnosed with metastatic malignant melanoma, a death sentence at that time. He underwent a 7-hour surgical procedure to remove his left sternocleidomastoid muscle, around which tumors had formed. After subsequent meetings with oncologists at Memorial Sloan Kettering left us hopeless about treatment, we turned to macrobiotics. And just when we had become salmon and seaweed skeletons, God led us to Dr Nick through a research organization recommended by a friend.

In his madras shirt and jeans, the handsome, energetic young man who greeted us in the waiting room was a stark contrast to the solemn white-haired doctors we'd previously met with. We knew Nick's protocol was individually diet based, and as we took seats in front of his desk, I jokingly said, "We're hoping you'll tell us Jerry can have a steak and baked potato when we get home."

Before our meeting, Jerry had blood work done and had sent in a hair sample. Flipping through Jerry's folder, Nick said, "Yes, a steak and baked potato would be good. But make sure you use plenty of butter and sour cream." He looked up and with twinkling, soul-piercing eyes, laser-beamed on Jerry as only Nick could. And he said something we never thought we'd hear: "I think you're going to be just fine."

That was 27 years ago. Like hundreds of others, my husband is alive, well, and thriving today because of Nicholas Gonzalez and his lifelong dedication to curing cancer and other degenerative diseases. Why he was taken from us is a question as wide as the wind. But I was comforted when I learned that Nick and his wife,

Mary Beth, had a strong Christian faith. Because I believe that Christ, the Great Physician Himself, had been Nick's ultimate mentor. And that when they met, Nick heard the words all of us hope to one day hear: "Well done, good and faithful servant!" (Matthew 25:21, New International Version).

Tribute to a Friend and Doctor

Suzanne Somers

It's my honor today to give tribute to my friend, my doctor, Nick Gonzalez. I also am here today with a heavy heart. He was a lone voice, he was a one of a kind, he was fearless. I used to e-mail him on a regular basis and it didn't matter what time I would e-mail him, I would get an answer back. I would say "Go to bed," because he was 3 hours ahead of me. I used to joke with him that he worked like he was running out of time. Today I'm feeling that that was rather ironic because maybe he knew, maybe he knew deep down. His work was so special and so controversial because he had a theory about cancer that was effective—that it could be managed for life just like diabetes.

When I first interviewed him I said, "That's all well and good but I'd really have to speak to some of your patients." He allowed me to speak, with their permission, to 17 of his stage IV patients, all of whom had been alive 10 years, 21 years, 12 years, 17 years. With each interview, I became a believer. Then recently at his funeral services and the reception that was following, I talked to person after person, realizing that I had been in a little church packed with terminal patients, all of whom had been alive for over 10 years—many of them well over 10 years. One man said, "I was diagnosed with stage IV lung cancer 27 years ago and I was given no hope by orthodox medicine. I've been on Dr Gonzalez's protocol ever since."

I heard these stories over and over again, and not only is it a personal loss for me as a friend to lose Nick Gonzalez, the man to whom I went to time and time again for answers, for issues that had come up that became controversial. He was so well versed in everything. I always felt very proud to present him to a constituency that might never have had the opportunity to learn from him. That's what he was, a teacher. He taught me about how to keep my body healthy. His protocol was not only for cancer but it was a recipe for life in a toxic world that is bringing everyone down, and through him I felt that I could survive the environment.

He took away my fear of cancer, which is probably the greatest gift that anybody ever could have given me, having had cancer once myself. I credit him with keeping me alive and educating me in a way that now that, he is gone, I realize if I continue his protocol, I can expect to stay in the superb health that I am in today. He was very, very special and he was married to the perfect woman, Mary Beth, who recognized that being married to a genius is difficult. She gave him the space to do the work that took so much of his time and so much time away from her. She allowed that with love because she knew what he had to offer to people.

I think that there are 2 ways that we are remembered in life, or or judged, depending. One is by our accomplishments and the other is by our character. His accomplishments don't need to be stated. We know how magnificent he was and what a genius mind he had and what he had to offer to so many patients, which is hope, who have lived because of their belief in him. The other part of Nick Gonzalez is his character. He was kind, he was humble, he was brilliant, he was a maverick. He fearlessly criticized the shortcomings of allopathic medicine. We are better off having had him on this planet. God bless you Nick. We will miss you. I will miss you. Humanity has had a great loss. Rest in peace.

Nicholas J. Gonzalez, MD, in Conversation With Peter Barry Chowka

This interview was conducted in Dr Gonzalez's office in New York, New York, on February 12, 2005.

Peter Barry Chowka: When and how did you first meet William Donald Kelley, DDS?[1,2]

Nicholas J. Gonzalez, MD: Through a writer friend of mine, I met Kelley one afternoon in July of 1981 in a chiropractor's office in Forest Hills, Queens, New York, after the completion of my second year of medical school.

Chowka: During that first encounter with Kelley, what kind of impression did he make on you?

Dr Gonzalez: Totally strong impression. Within 5 minutes I thought he was probably the smartest man I'd ever met. I was already working under Robert Good, MD, PhD, who was the president of Sloan-Kettering at the time and the most published author in the history of medicine.[3] And I'd already met a number of other eminent scientists, people like Linus Pauling, PhD[4]—and all of the bright people at Sloan-Kettering and the Rockefeller Institute. And Dr Kelley was so far above—just in terms of pure intelligence that came

out when you asked him the right questions. When I started talking to him about science, I immediately could see that not only was this man very serious but he had knowledge that one finds only in someone who is very, very smart. So, yes, within minutes I thought he was clearly one of the smartest people I would ever meet. I never changed that opinion.

I mentioned to Dr Kelley that I could talk to Dr Good about him. His eyes lit up and he said he'd followed Dr Good's career for years and he felt Dr Good was the only person in orthodox medicine with enough intelligence and enough of an open mind to take him seriously.

Later that afternoon, after leaving Dr Kelley, I went up to see Dr Good in his office, without an appointment. He was already mentoring me. We talked for about an hour about Dr Kelley and, based on what I told him about what I had just learned that afternoon, Dr Good said, "You know, unusual ideas don't always fit the mainstream model. Dr Kelley may be a fraud, but he also may be real, and you can never know. He's probably worthy of an investigation."

Dr Good really encouraged me to start investigating Kelley. The next day, I flew down to Dallas where Dr Kelley was living and had his office, and I started doing my project that would develop into a 5-year study, which I completed under Dr Good when I was doing my immunology fellowship training.

Chowka: At that point, 1981, what led you—a conventionally-trained medical student—to be interested in what someone like Dr Kelley had to offer, in that rather early period of nutritional medicine?

Dr Gonzalez: I didn't really think of it as nutritional medicine as much as a scientific issue. I guess I'm too stupid to be prejudiced [laughs]. It was a question of could he get patients well or not. I didn't really care whether he was alternative. Certain things he said rang so true scientifically that had nothing to do with alternative or nutritional or mainstream—they just seemed true. And that's the way I went forward with it.

I came out of a research background working with Dr Good where you looked for the brilliant new idea, not in the mainstream but in the fringe. Dr Good was a great medical historian. He knew that pioneering thinkers like Semmelweis had been totally ostracized and died in a mental institution. And Pasteur did some of his greatest work in a barn because the medical establishment hated him and actually tried to criminalize his work. Dr Good knew of the resistance to people like Lister and Galileo. So he was very anxious to investigate someone like Dr Kelley who was offbeat.

Chowka: At the point that you began to look into Dr Kelley, were any of your colleagues or associates at your level of medicine similarly oriented and open minded, or were you unique in that regard?

Dr Gonzalez: Most of the medical students were very conservative and believed whatever the professors told them.

Chowka: Why were you different—because you had been a journalist?

Dr Gonzalez: I came from a different background. First, I was older. I had been an investigative reporter. I had very good mentors when I was a journalist. My first editorial mentor at *Time-Life* was Byron Dobell, who had been managing editor of *Esquire*. He said if you go into any story with a preconceived notion of what's true, you're going to miss the truly great stories. You have to get rid of all of your prejudices and biases or you'll be a third-rate journalist and a fourth-rate writer, and you're going to miss some great stories. And that applied when I went to medical school in terms of science. I never accepted what was told to me as true. I wasn't a rebel in the sense that I accepted that it *wasn't* true. I just never accepted it as true. So when something unusual crossed my path, like Dr Kelley, I was perfectly willing to accept it without a second thought. I was willing to give Dr Kelley the benefit of the doubt.

Chowka: How long, after you started in 1981 to put the research project together, did you continue to work with or around Dr Kelley?

Dr Gonzalez: I had to finish medical school and do my internship. At the end of my internship, Dr Good asked me to join his group as a full-time fellow. He was pushed out of Sloan-Kettering and he went on this journey across America. He spent a year at the University of Oklahoma setting up a cancer research division, and then he went to the University of South Florida. I followed him to Oklahoma and then to Florida for 2 years after I finished my internship, basically doing nothing but my Kelley investigation. He provided funding, the resources, the facilities, a salary, and basically encouraged me 100% to do this. And that's what I did. He thought it was important enough to support that.

Chowka: In order to maintain that support, financially and otherwise, did you have to write proposals, or be approved by boards or something?

Dr Gonzalez: Dr Robert Good was powerful enough. He got me a salary. I have never filled out a grant proposal. I got Dr Good to support me and the funding came strictly from his word, verbal word.

Chowka: Would such a thing be possible today?

Dr Gonzalez: We got the grant in 1993 from Nestlé for our first pilot study.[5] It was done over dinner. I never filled out a grant proposal. Just Dr [Pierre] Guesry's word. He was chief of research at Nestlé.

Chowka: It seems fairly novel, that that kind of thing can still happen.

Dr Gonzalez: [Laughs] Yes, so I've been told. I don't say this boastfully; you asked me a factual question. I don't mean to be self-serving at all. The NCCAM grant[6] also was approved without a grant proposal.

Chowka: Because of the pilot study?

Dr Gonzalez: Based on the pilot study. In 1999, I had a meeting with Richard Klausner, MD, who was the head of the National Cancer Institute, in Rep. Dan Burton's office. Klausner's attitude was based on the pilot study's results: *This needed to be funded.* He said right there, "It's funded." And we never had to fill out a formal grant proposal. The fact is I've never written a grant proposal in my life. And Proctor and Gamble, too—they put in $5 million in research funding during the 3-year period when we worked together. And they just did it, based on what they believed in terms of my work.

Chowka: So you did it your way.

Dr Gonzalez: I did it my way, yeah—as the *New Yorker*[7] piece said, I come from a family of people who do it their own way. My grandfather, the cellist, was also a revolutionary who, at the height of his career at age 21, decided to go into the mountains with Pancho Villa to fight for democracy in Mexico, which was a losing proposition then and now. His side was basically decimated during the first years of the revolution. With a price on his head, he had to leave the country. He escaped Mexico with his cello and his wife and nothing else—and he came to New York as a refugee. So I come from a family that kind of does things their own way.

Chowka: Back to the early 1980s when you were studying Dr Kelley's work, what was he like to work with? You were the first qualified, research-oriented person to take a serious interest in his work.

Dr Gonzalez: It wasn't what I was used to, at the austere, refined atmosphere of Sloan-Kettering. Within about a week of arriving in Dallas, I said to Dr Kelley, "You know, it looks like every crazy in America somehow makes his way into your office." His office in Dallas was a frenetic center of total chaos. It was just this nonstop parade of people coming into his office wanting something from him. I'd never seen anything like it.

Chowka: That sounds a lot like Mildred Nelson, RN's office at the Bio-Medical Center (Hoxsey therapy) clinic in Tijuana during her heyday when I would spend hours there observing her work.[8] There were no doors on her office. It was wide open, people just walked in. If you stood or sat there long enough, you'd get an audience with her. All kinds of pitch men kept coming in.

Dr Gonzalez: There was a lot of that in Dallas. It's interesting: I've learned that when someone has the truth, it attracts everybody, from every background, for every possible motivation—good, bad, noble, evil, and indifferent. People went to Dr Kelley because they thought he was like a guru; he had this magical ability to cure people. There were people who wanted to steal his work, people who wanted to sell his work, and people who saw him as nothing more than a way to make a lot of money.

Chowka: Did he entertain all of these people equally, without prejudice? Did he throw some of them out?

Dr Gonzalez: No, he never threw anybody out. In fact, I started throwing people out because it was interfering with our work. And I was actually living in his apartment at that point. I was willing to stay in a hotel. He said, "Stay in my apartment." It was a very modest, 1-bedroom apartment on the outskirts of Dallas near his office. One of his daughters lived there and they made me take the bedroom. Kelley slept on the couch, [and] his daughter slept on the floor. Dr Kelley and I spent a lot of time together there. That's when I really began to ask him about his work. Neither he nor I needed a lot of sleep, so we talked for hours every evening in his apartment when it was quiet.

I spent a number of weeks there. I was able to really get down to work and to gather together a whole series of charts of his patients who seemed to have appropriately diagnosed biopsy proven cancer that by anybody's orthodox standards got better.

Chowka: And these patients had been treated by Dr Kelley directly?

Dr Gonzalez: Both by him and by some of his counselors using the Kelley therapy.

Chowka: During what period?

Dr Gonzalez: Starting in the early 1970s to that time, 1981.

Chowka: So these were, in effect, his best cases?

Dr Gonzalez: It was basically the first best case series ever done for an alternative therapy. I was working 14-hour days that first time in Dallas. I put together records, interviewed the patients, made sure they were real, started getting their medical records, put them in a suitcase, went back to Sloan-Kettering, and met with Dr Good for a period of several days.

Dr Good said that the outcomes of the cases I was showing him went beyond anything he had ever seen in all his years as a cancer expert at the top of the profession. And he said this really warranted a serious investigation, which I continued even through third-year medical school. And then when I was a fourth-year medical student, I got permission to spend 4 months doing independent research under Dr Good to investigate Dr Kelley. That's when I went up to Winthrop, Washington, and actually lived in Dr Kelley's house there. He had about 10 000 records in Winthrop. That's where his main body of records was.

Chowka: What was your model for how you went ahead in evaluating Dr Kelley's results at this point? As you said, it was in effect the first test of its kind. Did you make it up as you went?

Dr Gonzalez: We didn't make it up. I spent a lot of time in Dr Good's office discussing how to approach this, because basically we were dealing with a practitioner who wasn't in the orthodox medical world and not with a controlled clinical trial situation. Dr Good said, you still can get good data from this. He knew about Gerson's book.[9] He suggested I should put together a series of 50 patients with a variety of different cancers treated by Dr Kelley who had been appropriately diagnosed with biopsies and who clearly had done well. He said that will give us some idea whether he treats a variety of cancers successfully. He said that's not going to be helpful in determining what Dr Kelley's success rate is, because these are his best cases. So what you need is the records of all of the patients who entered Kelley's office in a specified period of time diagnosed with pancreatic cancer and find out what happened to them. Dr Good suggested pancreatic cancer because it is the worst cancer in terms of survival.

Dr Kelley immediately jumped at the idea. That's one of the reasons I always respected Kelley—we were asking him to open up his charts, show us what he could do with the worst cancer there is—it really put him in a very vulnerable situation. I guarantee there are very few orthodox physicians who would put their careers on the line based on their success with pancreatic cancer. And Dr Kelley didn't hesitate. He said, "Great!" In fact, that's exactly what he said: "Great!" He said, "Let's do it."

Chowka: Dr Good sounds like the key person in getting everything going. He really helped to facilitate it.

Dr Gonzalez: Totally. Without Dr Good, it never would have happened. Period. After my internship, I joined Dr Good and that's when I had the full time to continue the Kelley project. Without Dr Good I would have just continued on the orthodox route, gone through my residency, hated it, and just become another orthodox researcher. Without Dr Good, there never would have been a best case series of Dr Kelley, there never would have been that first monograph,[10] I

never would have had the opportunity to learn Dr Kelley's work, in time. It was about 1985 when Dr Kelley started having seizures that really changed him, both in personality and motivation. And he became more difficult to work with. By 1987, it was so difficult to work with him that I just broke off and I never spoke to him again.

Chowka: What were the seizures about?

Dr Gonzalez: After I met Dr Kelley, he started having very serious atrial fibrillation and cardiac arrhythmias, and I think that's what precipitated the seizures. When the heart doesn't beat properly, you don't get enough blood to the brain and you can end up with seizures. He had a series of grand mal seizures. As eccentric as he was before, and certainly you knew him very well in the 1980s, he became almost impossibly difficult after that series of seizures. Had Dr Good not encouraged me to start my investigation when I did, Dr Kelley would have never been sound enough for me to do the study properly.

So I had about 5 glory years when Dr Kelley was sharp—especially when I lived with him in Winthrop, Washington, at his farm; I was there for 4 months without a break. All extraneous distractions were eliminated. We lived organically, we lived off the farm food—it was all organic. We just concentrated on the work. And he was as sharp as could be.

Chowka: He was giving a lot of time to the project?

Dr Gonzalez: He gave full time to it. He said this is the most important thing he could ever do. He thought that working with me, under Dr Good, was like some dream come true. He said this is his one opportunity to get his work properly tested and evaluated

Chowka: Did Good ever communicate with Dr Kelley?

Dr Gonzalez: Yes, in fact we all had dinner together once, in Oklahoma City. Dr Good wanted to meet him. So Dr Kelley came up from Dallas. Dr Good and his girlfriend and Dr Kelley and I had dinner at a Vietnamese restaurant in Oklahoma City.

Chowka: Both you and I got a strong, positive impression of Dr Kelley on first meeting him— here's a man who is very bright, very sincere, well-motivated, a humanitarian. Does the fact that he was a special quote/unquote individual in that regard maybe have an impact on the clinical results he or anyone so motivated would get?

Dr Gonzalez: All that's true. Very few people were as smart as Dr Kelley. They just didn't know as much as he knew. This is a guy who had spent 30 years studying nutrition and he knew it from top to bottom. His library in Winthrop, with 10 000 volumes—esoteric nutrition books I didn't even know existed. That's where I first saw Beard's book[11] on Dr Kelley's bookshelf.

Chowka: But you also mentioned that in Dallas he lived simply.

Dr Gonzalez: Yes.

Chowka: He was not into accumulating.

Dr Gonzalez: Oh, no, no, no. He had nothing. People think that he did it for the money. What are they, crazy? He could have made $5 million a year as an orthodontist. This is a guy who had nothing.

You've asked a lot of questions— could other people do the therapy is essentially what you're asking. Dr Kelley had this unique ability: He was an instinctive healer, you hear about people like that—doctors that are just smarter than other doctors, and they have a greater instinct for healing.

Chowka: And they can help to motivate their patients.

Dr Gonzalez: Totally, and he did. And his patients loved him. I interviewed more than a thousand of his patients. Some of them I interviewed multiple times. Some of his patients I interviewed 6 or 8 times. Some of them I actually visited them in their homes. And they all loved him. They would do anything for him, to help him, to defend him. He'd saved their lives. They were extraordinary stories, the most moving stories I'd ever heard.

Chowka: I want to focus on this question about the individuals who are special healers. Is there something else going on with them that really helped them to reach the patient? In my experience of observing and reporting on remarkable healers, ultimately a great degree of their effectiveness—and it's impossible to quantify, of course—seems to come down to inspiring and motivating the patient to get well based on establishing a real connection with the patient. I spent a lot of time with Mildred Nelson, RN, not to the extent that you did with Dr Kelley, but I had the chance to observe her for more than 19 years, sometimes for weeks at a time. I saw her treat many, many patients with the Hoxsey therapy. She had this unique ability to individualize or tailor her clinical approach to her patients, spontaneously, depending on what she thought or felt they needed. Did the patient need a firm hand, or did he or she require a soft touch and a supportive shoulder to cry on—very individually tailoring the psychological dimension of the treatment to that patient in that moment.

Dr Gonzalez: The sad thing is that's the kind of manner and ability that every doctor should have. What's tragic is that it's rare. What Dr Kelley did should be typical. That's what doctors should be trained to do. And they're not. In that respect, Dr Kelley was very unusual. He immediately developed a rapport with his patients, and they loved him and he motivated them so they would do the therapy. And that's

critical, especially with a lifestyle program like his. This isn't like chemotherapy, where it doesn't matter if you like the doctor, or if you even see the doctor, you just stick out your arm and eat ice cream and watch some stupid TV while you're getting chemo.

Chowka: And zone out while you're getting the chemotherapy.

Dr Gonzalez: In fact they want you to zone out! They don't want you to question, or to think too much, or to read books. They want you to zone out, eat ice cream, keep your weight up, and put your arm out so the nurse can give you the chemo. Don't ask questions. You ask questions, you're going to cause trouble for the oncologist.

It's not some kind of mystical quality that only Dr Kelley or Mildred Nelson had. But the way they were is the way that it should be.

Chowka: It's traditional.

Dr Gonzalez: Yes, it should be the way doctors are trained. And if a person in medical training doesn't have that kind of personality, he should be booted out. But of course medical schools really gear themselves for the exact opposite of that—for very aggressive, ambitious people who work their butts off to get into medical school. It's not about taking care of patients or developing these kinds of interpersonal skills. It's about competition and being the best and being the smartest and getting the highest medical board scores because otherwise you won't get into the right medical school and all that other kind of stuff. Actually taking care of patients has nothing to do with that at all. It has nothing to do with creativity, either.

Chowka: To sort of wrap Dr Kelley up with a bow: In the history of what we're talking about here, not only alternative medicine but medicine itself, how do you see him and his legacy at this point?

Dr Gonzalez: I think someday Dr Kelley is going to be viewed as one of the great pioneers in medicine. His work will be the foundation for a new medicine that's scientifically verifiable, that has a strong scientific base, that stands up to clinical work, to clinical trials, even to animal studies, and that can be transferred [replicated]. You know Linda Isaacs, MD, and I are getting results as good as Dr Kelley. It's not that I'm trying to beat my own drum—if we didn't, if we got only some people well, I'd be happy. But we know what happens to every single patient that enters our office, and I know what happened to Dr Kelley's patients during a 15-year period.

Chowka: To clarify that—you see your work clinically as coming from or in a lineage that started with Dr Kelley?

Dr Gonzalez: Yes, we use the enzymes as he did and we use his concepts of autonomic dominance in our work. That's how we approach patients. Dr Kelley's work isn't something he developed himself. Beard published his first paper in *The Lancet* about the enzymes and their anticancer effect in 1902. The Krebses, eccentric as they were, during the 1940s rediscovered Beard. And the whole concept of sympathetic/parasympathetic dominance goes back to Francis Pottenger, MD—one of the great neuroscientists of the first half of the 20th century. His real contribution was in autonomic physiology, and he wrote a classic textbook, *Symptoms of Visceral Disease*,[12] which gave Dr Kelley the insights to develop his whole autonomic/sympathetic/parasympathetic paradigm.

So Dr Kelley comes from a lineage of other people, even going back to Pavlov. Pavlov was actually an expert in the autonomic nervous system. A lot of Dr Pottenger's work came out of what Pavlov was doing. Pavlov thought that some people had a strong sympathetic system, and other people had a strong parasympathetic system. So Dr Kelley's own sophisticated work with autonomic physiology goes back to other people. That's not an attempt to diminish Dr Kelley. In fact, it makes him even more sound.

Chowka: I see that kind of thing as enhancing one's argument or impact. As a journalist, I've always felt that it strengthens a writer's case when you can cite or build on other's work, both contemporaries and those who have come before. There's nobody who springs forth with all of the answers. But in today's world, especially, that's how most people try to present themselves.

Dr Gonzalez: Yes, that's right. Beard published papers in the major medical journals during the first decade of the 20th century, reporting cases with advanced, appropriately diagnosed, biopsy-proven cancer that had total regression using enzymes. These cases go back 100 years now. And yes, 100 years ago they knew how to diagnose cancer and they knew how to read pathology slides and they were very sophisticated about diagnosing—and they could break it down into the different types of breast cancer and different types of colon cancer. They knew how to do it. And these patients clearly had cancer and they were verified by experts at major academic institutions, both in the United States and in Europe. I have records of case after case of patients successfully treated 100 years ago with injectable enzymes.

So the fact that there's a history only makes the case stronger. In fact, that's one of the first things that impressed me during my first 5 minutes with Dr Kelley—he very quickly started talking about other people, like Beard and Pottenger, rather than himself. I said: Whoa, there's actually a history to this. When he started talking about the details of the placenta it made a lot of sense. I asked him, "Is this your work?" He said, "No, Beard actually was the first person." There was a lot of humility to Dr Kelley. Even though it was his therapy, he was already giving credit to other people. That impressed me.

To sum up, to get back to your question, I think Dr Kelley will be appreciated someday as one of the great innovators in medicine. I think he really will be seen as one of the people laying down a foundation for a very productive, new model of medicine. I think all his foibles and eccentricities will be forgotten. And what we will remember is how brilliant he was, which is how I remember him.

Chowka: I'm in the city this week for a big CAM expo at the Grand Hyatt New York, which, ironically, is where I first met Dr Kelley 25 years ago at an alternative cancer conference. In recent years, the name CAM—complementary alternative medicine—has always rubbed me the wrong way because "complementary" suggests, obviously, that it's a complement or an adjunct to mainstream or conventional medicine. Your therapy is a primary therapy. That was the case with most of the original alternative cancer therapy pioneers. There don't seem to be many primary alternative cancer therapies left today.

Dr Gonzalez: What you're saying is absolutely true. But complementary is what a lot of alternative doctors want to be, because they don't have the guts or the ability to take it on as a primary therapy.

I make it clear that what we do clinically is not complementary—this is a primary cancer treatment. Period. That's what it is. It's not anything else. And that makes a lot of people nervous. My greatest opposition has often come from within the so-called alternative world. We've made it clear that first we have to prove that our therapy works and write the book about it so that scientists can read it and learn the basics. And then we'll start training people. We're not going to start training people *first* and then prove the therapy; we're going to do it the way it should be done.

Chowka: What would you like to see your work lead to, or what kind of effect do you hope that it has?

Dr Gonzalez: My wish is that my work will do several things. First, show that what we do is based on real science—the enzyme part, Beard's work, even the autonomic physiology part—all based on science. And show how Dr Kelley's concepts about autonomic dominance are absolutely, totally accurate. So I want that to be established. And, with that, get scientists and doctors and lay people to start thinking that this really is not just some other kind of cancer therapy but maybe a new model of medicine that might be very valid. The third part is to generate a lot of discussion. We may not change the course of medicine, which was Dr Kelley's goal. But at least we'll get the issues out there so people can discuss them more intelligently. Right now, there's a vacuum of information.

REFERENCES

1. Chowka PB. Steve McQueen: Legacy of a medical outlaw. *New Age.* 1981;6(7):28-37.
2. Rohé F. *Metabolic Ecology: A Way To Win The Cancer War.* Winfield, KS: Wedgestone Press; 1981.
3. Cooper MD. Robert A. Good, May 21, 1922-June 13, 2003. *J Immunol.* 2003;171(12):6318-6319.
4. Chowka PB. Linus Pauling, PhD: The last interview. *Nutr Sci News.* 1996;1:26-28.
5. Gonzalez NJ, Isaacs LL. Evaluation of pancreatic proteolytic enzyme treatment of adenocarcinoma of the pancreas, with nutrition and detoxification support. *Nutr Cancer.* 1999;33(2);117-124.
6. Chowka PB. One man alone. *Altern Med.* 2002;47:56-67.
7. Specter M. The outlaw doctor. *The New Yorker.* February 5, 2001:48-61.
8. Chowka PB. Does Mildred Nelson have a cure for cancer? In: Moffet J, ed. *Points of Departure: An Anthology of Non-Fiction.* New York, NY: New American Library; 1985:302-311.
9. Gerson, M. *A Cancer Therapy: Results of Fifty Cases.* New York, NY: Whittier Books; 1958.
10. Gonzalez N. *One Man, Alone: An Investigation of Nutrition, Cancer, and William Donald Kelley.* New York, NY: New Spring Press; 2010.
11. Beard J. *The Enzyme Treatment of Cancer and Its Scientific Basis.* London, United Kingdom: Chatto and Windus; 1911.
12. Pottenger FM. *Symptoms of Visceral Disease.* 5th ed. Saint Louis, MO: The C.V. Mosby Co; 1938.

The History of the Gonzalez Cancer Treatment Model

Colin A. Ross, MD

The treatment protocol developed by Nicholas Gonzalez, MD, has its origins in the work of John Beard, DSc,[1-4] in the early 20th century. Dr Beard was an embryologist and histologist who made a number of original discoveries and who was nominated for a Nobel Prize. He was the first to identify adult stem cells, a codiscoverer of Rohon-Beard cells in the spinal cord, the first to describe cell apoptosis, the first to describe the immune functions of the thymus, and the first to state that the corpus luteum inhibits ovulation during pregnancy. All of these discoveries were based on his study of thousands of slides he prepared from embryos from many different species.

In the course of his studies, Beard focused his attention on the trophoblast, which is the precursor of the placenta. The trophoblast must invade the wall of the uterus, and anchor in it, for the fetus to survive. Early in the pregnancy, the trophoblast cells have the following properties: (1) undifferentiated, invasive, migratory, and angiogenic (create their own blood supply); (2) resistant to immune surveillance; and (3) lack normal cell adhesion. The cells have to have these properties to carry out their functions. For instance, if trophoblasts could not resist immune surveillance, the mother's immune system would recognize the paternal antigens in their cell membranes, a host-versus-graft reaction would be set up, the mother would reject the fetus, and the fetus would die. If trophoblasts were not angiogenic, they would not receive enough oxygen and nutrients to carry out their functions.

In normal fetal development, the trophoblast transforms into the stable placenta. Placental cells are differentiated, noninvasive, nonangiogenic, and have normal cell adhesion. If the trophoblast does not convert to a stable placenta, a choriocarcinoma develops; the cancer invades through the wall of the uterus and kills the mother.

While studying the trophoblast, Beard observed that approximately 15% of trophoblast cells are distributed throughout the body, where they remain in a dormant state. He called these cells *wayward trophoblasts*. In modern terminology, these wayward trophoblasts are *adult stem cells*. Beard also observed that the time in fetal development when the trophoblast transforms into the stable placenta is the same period that the fetal pancreas begins secreting pancreatic enzymes, principally trypsin and amylase. He called amylase, *amylopsin*, but it is the same molecule that we now call *amylase*.

The next step in Beard's thinking was his hypothesis that pancreatic enzymes are the signal that converts the trophoblast into the placenta. Up to this point, Beard was not thinking about cancer at all. The next, and revolutionary step, occurred when Beard hypothesized 2 things: (1) cancer arises from wayward trophoblasts that have escaped normal regulatory control, and (2) pancreatic enzymes could be used to treat cancer.

Step 2 was based on Beard's realization that the properties of normal trophoblasts and cancer cells are the same: They are undifferentiated, invasive, angiogenic, migratory, resistant to immune surveillance, and lack normal cell adhesion. According to Beard's theory, cancer cells are not normal cells that have dedifferentiated backward in the direction of stem cells. Rather, they are wayward trophoblasts that have escaped normal regulatory control, and they have taken on some of the features of their surrounding tissue due to local signaling in that tissue. Thus, trophoblasts that escape control in the breast look like dedifferentiated breast cells, and the same for brain, muscle, and all other tissues. Pancreatic enzymes, then, can potentially convert many different cancers back into stable cells that do not invade and kill their host, because the cancer cells are trophoblasts that are normally stabilized by pancreatic enzymes.

There are many additional details to the Beard theory that are described elsewhere.[4,5] Early in the 20th century, Beard began treating cancer with pancreatic enzymes, with some spectacular responses. Other doctors around the globe began using these enzymes as a treatment for cancer, but a number of problems arose, including doctors prescribing insufficient doses or using improperly prepared and inert enzymes. After a couple of decades, the use of pancreatic enzymes for the treatment of cancer disappeared.

Then, in the 1950s, a Fort Worth dentist named Donald Kelley[6] read about John Beard, and he began to experiment with the treatment of cancer using pancreatic enzymes. He developed a treatment protocol that involved intensive nutritional support with diet and supplements, as well as a primary active treatment with pancreatic enzymes. He had many remarkable and successful outcomes in cases of advanced cancer, with survivals much longer than those obtained with conventional surgery, radiation, and chemotherapy.

Dr Nicholas Gonzalez heard about Dr Kelley's work while a medical resident. He travelled to Fort Worth, met with Kelley, studied a large series of his cases, and decided to begin treating cancer with pancreatic enzymes himself. This eventually lead to his setting up a private practice in New York and partnering with Linda Isaacs, MD, who has continued the treatment after Dr Gonzalez's sudden death on July 21, 2015.

The treatment of cancer with pancreatic enzymes has not been accepted by mainstream medicine, although it has received considerable publicity[7] and has been validated in a pilot study with human patients[8] and in an animal study.[9] Why is this? One reason is that there is not a sufficient body of replicated research to prove the effectiveness of the treatment regimen to physicians and scientists. Therefore, the treatment can be dismissed as unproven, anecdotal, "experimental," or unscientific.

But think about it for a minute. What if a doctor discovered a supplement that can regenerate brain cells? If that doctor published a single, fully documented case in which a person were shot in the head with massive, fatal brain damage, demonstrated on MRI, but was then kept on life support, given the supplement, and regrew a normal brain, woke up out of coma, and was cognitively intact with normal motor and sensory function, how would the medical world react? It would take only 1 case. Money would be poured into studying this revolutionary, life-saving treatment. We would not be hearing statements about anecdote, spontaneous remission, selection bias, or fraud—all accusations that have been directed at Dr Gonzalez.

Of course, further research, study, and replication would be required. What if this doctor had a series of more than 100 such cases, as Dr Gonzalez has? What would the reaction be then? So, why has the treatment of cancer with pancreatic enzymes been ignored by most of medicine, when it can be equally as life-saving? I think there are several explanations. First, there is a paradigm shift problem: There is always institutionalized resistance to any paradigm shift. A recent example is the resistance mounted by organized medicine to accepting that many stomach ulcers are caused not by excess acid, but by an easily treated bacterial infection. This discovery was discredited and marginalized initially, but it is now common knowledge.

Another force at play is the fact that pancreatic enzymes cannot be patented because they occur naturally. That means that there is no drug company money being invested in them. Third, the treatment regimen is regarded as a form of complementary or alternative medicine at present, which means that it has to overcome substantial resistance from mainstream medicine.

Another factor at work is the National Cancer Institute (NCI)-funded study of the treatment of pancreatic cancer with pancreatic enzymes versus standard chemotherapy with gemcitabine.[10,11] This study, which was run by oncologists at Columbia, reported that the average survival time for patients treated with gemcitabine was 14 months, whereas the average survival time for patients treated with pancreatic enzymes was 4.3 months.[10] Taken at face value, these results indicate that the Gonzalez regimen is not worthy of further research funding or study, and it should be abandoned.

There are so many severe methodological problems with this study, however, that it should be disregarded, and, I would say, formally retracted by the editor of the journal in which it was published.[11,12] Of 39 patients assigned to the pancreatic enzyme arm of the study, only 1 followed the protocol completely. Thirty either did not take any enzymes at all, or they took them incompletely or for short periods. This is equivalent to a study that finds that 2 mg of aspirin has no effect. What would we conclude from such a study? We would conclude that the results are meaningless and tell us nothing about the effectiveness of aspirin.

Why, then, can such a study get published, and get endorsed on the NCI Web site as authoritative?[i] The nonacceptance of the Gonzalez regimen cannot be explained by good medical practice, healthy skepticism, or anything of the sort. The treatment outcomes attainable with the Gonzalez regimen are life-saving in many cases and consist of good quality of life for years or decades beyond the average survival times with standard medical treatment.

This, then, is the history of the Gonzalez cancer treatment model. The model could well disappear again, as it did 100 years ago. The purpose of this special book by the publoshers of *Alternative Therapies in Health and Medicine* is to help ward off that outcome. The treatment outcomes obtained with the Gonzalez regimen are something that should be accepted and validated by mainstream medicine. Substantial resources should be allocated to studying the trophoblast model of cancer at many different levels, from genetics and biochemistry; through cell biology, physiology, embryology, and pharmacology; to clinical oncology.

REFERENCES

1. Beard J. *The Enzyme Treatment of Cancer and its Scientific Basis*. New York, NY: New Spring Press; 2010.
2. Moss RW. Enzymes, trophoblasts, and cancer: The afterlife of an idea (1924–2008). *Integr Cancer Ther*. 2008;7(4):262-275.
3. Moss RW. The life and times of John Beard, DSc (1858–1924). *Integr Cancer Ther*. 2008;7(4):229-251.
4. Ross CA. The trophoblast model of cancer. *Nut Cancer*. 2015;67(1):61-67.
5. Gonzalez NJ, Isaacs LL. *The Trophoblast and the Origins of Cancer: One Solution to the Medical Enigma of our Time*. New York, NY: New Spring Press; 2009.
6. Gonzalez NJ. *One Man Alone. An Investigation of Nutrition, Cancer and William Donald Kelley*. New York, NY: New Spring Press; 2010.
7. Somers S. *Knockout: Interviews with Doctors Who Are Curing Cancer—And How to Prevent Getting It in the First Place*. New York, NY: Three Rivers Press; 2010.
8. Gonzalez NJ, Isaacs, LL. Evaluation of pancreatic enzyme proteolytic enzyme treatment of adenocarcinoma of the pancreas. *Nutr Cancer*. 1999;33(2):117-124.
9. Saruc R, Standop S, Nozawa F, et al. Pancreatic enzyme extract improves survival in murine pancreatic cancer. *Pancreas*. 2004;28(4):401-412.
10. Chabot JA, Tsai WY, Fine RL, et al. Pancreatic proteolytic enzyme therapy compared with gemcitabine-based chemotherapy for the treatment of pancreatic cancer. *J Clin Oncol*. 2010;28(12):2058-2063.
11. Ross CA. Methodological flaws in the Chabot trial of pancreatic enzymes for the treatment of pancreatic cancer. *Int J Cancer Prev Res*. 2015;1:1-4.
12. Gonzalez NJ. *What Went Wrong? The Truth Behind the Clinical Trial of the Enzyme Treatment of Cancer*. New York, NY: New Spring Press; 2012.

i. See http://www.cancer.gov/about-cancer/treatment/cam/hp/gonzalez-pdq

A Case of Insulin-dependent Diabetes

Nicholas Gonzalez, MD

The treatment of cancer with pancreatic enzymes according to the Gonzalez protocol has been well described,[1-3] as has the trophoblast model of cancer on which the protocol is based.[3] A trial of gemcitabine versus pancreatic enzymes for the treatment of pancreatic enzymes[4] is so flawed methodologically that its findings, which suggest that the Gonzalez protocol is ineffective for pancreatic cancer, should be ignored.[5,6] Gonzalez and Isaacs have reported individual cases and a small case series in which patients with advanced, magnetic resonance imaging (MRI) and biopsy-confirmed pancreatic cancer have had remarkably long survival times, often exceeding a decade.[1,3,5]

To date, however, the use of the Gonzalez protocol for medical problems other than cancer has not been reported. The purpose of this case report is to describe the case of a man with insulin-dependent diabetes, extreme fatigue and insomnia, paresthesias, and a host of other symptoms, who improved dramatically on the Gonzalez protocol.

CASE REPORT

Patient G is a 44-year-old white male medical device salesman from the northeast who first presented for consultation in late June, 2011. Family history was notable for: paternal grandmother with fatal myeloma; paternal grandfather, a smoker, with fatal lung cancer; and a paternal uncle with fatal liver cancer. Multiple family members had been diagnosed with hypertension. At the time Patient G first presented, his mother was being treated for adult onset noninsulin dependent diabetes, whereas his maternal grandmother had developed the insulin dependent form of the disease as an adult.

Patient G presented with a complicated history during the 4 years previous to his first consultation, though the genesis of his problems seemed to have occurred much earlier. A serious athlete in college, he played hockey, ran track, and lifted weights regularly. After graduation, he continued playing "aggressive" contact hockey in a local adult league. During a game in 2007, he experienced a serious fall and injury around the net, twisting his back as he fell and immediately developing "excruciating" lower back pain. The pain persisted for some 4 weeks during which time he was unable to work full time. When his situation did not improve, he consulted with his primary care physician, who arranged for an extensive diagnostic workup complete with a computed tomography (CT) scan of the abdomen as well as colonoscopy. All testing was within normal limits. Eventually, when his pain improved and he was able to resume his vigorous work schedule, he assumed the problem was resolved.

In June, 2008, 1 year after his accident, Patient G's general health suddenly worsened in a period of several weeks; he developed persistent, chronic fatigue that he would describe later as "incredible fatigue all the time." His eyes felt heavy, and his muscles, in all muscle groups, became uncharacteristically weak, which for this weight lifter was an unusual circumstance.

When the symptoms persisted, Patient G returned to his primary care physician who ordered blood studies that came back within normal limits except for a slightly elevated thyroid-stimulating hormone (TSH), thought to be due to an autoimmune thyroiditis. Lyme and a variety of other infectious markers were all negative. Patient G's physician prescribed levothyroxine for the hypothyroidism but suggested no other treatment at the time.

Despite the thyroid supplementation, Patient G's severe fatigue persisted, though he "pushed" himself through his work and forced himself to continue his vigorous exercise regimen. However, his work, which demanded increasingly long hours each day and standing for hours in operating rooms, became increasingly difficult to sustain.

By July 2008, Patient G was falling asleep easily during the day, while experiencing what he would describe to me as "brain cloudiness or fog." To complicate the situation he developed persistent, "terrible" insomnia, as well as episodes of anxiety and obsessive worrisome thoughts. All the while, his muscle weakness continued to worsen.

Through his own contacts he learned about a well-known internist at Hahnemann Medical College in Philadelphia known to handle "difficult" and enigmatic cases, who could be seen only by referral, which Patient G's primary care physician provided. After an initial consultation at Hahnemann, this physician began an intensive workup, checking for all manner of common as well as rare illnesses. The testing revealed a single abnormality, an elevation in acetylcholine receptor antibodies indicating possible myasthenia gravis. With that finding, Patient G then underwent continued evaluation at Hahnemann including muscle resistance testing, which was negative; a CT scan of the chest to rule out thymoma, (also negative); and endoscopy to check esophageal function, which proved to be normal. A multifiber electromyography (EMG) to assess muscle firing activity in patients with presumed myasthenia gravis revealed no abnormality consistent with the disease. Importantly, in terms of what would eventually play out, his blood sugars throughout this period were all within the normal range.

Despite the negative results, the Hahnemann physician decided, because of the borderline acetylcholine receptor antibodies, to start a course of the antcholinesterase pyridostigmine, the standard treatment for myasthenia. Patient G dutifully took the medication for 3 weeks but discontinued the drug when he could see no positive effect.

As he continued to deteriorate, Patient G took a leave of absence from work to concentrate on finding a solution to his condition. At that point, his insomnia had progressed to such a degree that his primary care physician prescribed zolpidem. With growing frustration at the lack of answers, on his own he decided to consult at the Myasthenia Gravis Specialty Center at Jefferson Medical College in Philadelphia. There, a single fiber EMG test, the most sensitive for neuromuscular disorder, showed nothing, so the doctors ruled out myasthenia as a diagnosis. Instead, deciding his whole problem to be psychological in nature, they referred him for psychiatric evaluation and treatment. Desperate for any solution, Patient G agreed to the plan and subsequently, as he would later tell me, he was prescribed "every different antidepressive medication on the market," none of which led to improvement in any of his symptoms and most of which left him feeling much worse.

Through sheer dint of will, he returned to work, though he experienced relentless exhaustion complicated by the continuing insomnia unresponsive to sleep medication. His muscles throughout his body chronically ached and he felt perpetually weak. He reported that during this time he was constantly "miserable from not being able to get any answers about my condition." Though depressed, he felt more anger than depression because no one had any solution to his situation.

In January 2009, for the first time he developed daily severe headaches, but nonetheless he continued pushing himself in his work. In frustration, he then decided to consult with a local neurologist who did extensive titers for Lyme and other infectious agents. This physician ruled out myasthenia, but despite the negative antibodies the physician decided that Patient G's problems were due to Lyme disease. After placement of an intravenous (IV) port, Patient G began a 6-week course of IV high-dose ceftriaxone, learning to administer the antibiotic himself at home and even on the job so he could continue working. But at the end of the 6 weeks, he experienced no improvement; in fact, he felt only worse.

By September, 2009, he had deteriorated to such a degree that he could no longer work. December 2009 proved to be a particularly difficult time for him, to the point that he began feeling he might be dying because of the severity of his muscle weakness, fatigue, and diffuse muscle pain. In desperation he began looking into unconventional medical approaches, eventually consulting with a well-known alternative physician in New Jersey whom he found open minded and sincerely concerned about his situation. This physician once again raised the issue of myasthenia gravis because of the persistent muscle pain and weakness, though extensive blood testing this time around revealed only borderline positive Lyme titers. The physician started Patient G on an intensive supplement program and then admitted him to a local hospital for 3 days of intensive antibiotic treatment.

After completing the course of IV antibiotics, Patient G was discharged with plans for him to continue oral antibiotics. Despite the therapy, he would experience "absolutely no improvement" in any of his symptoms.

Nonetheless, Patient G continued under the care of this alternative physician for 3 months before discontinuing the relationship because of his lack of improvement and his ongoing decline. During this period, he developed new symptoms, including eyelid twitching and bags under his eyes so severe that it appeared, as he would later report, that he had swollen cheeks. His hands began to "shake" with tremors; he developed severe burning pain bilaterally in his feet; and he rapidly lost all the hair on his arms, legs, and chest, and even his eyebrows began to thin. In addition, he developed acute onset severe periodontal disease and potency issues.

He then decided to consult with another well-known alternative practitioner in New Jersey, who prescribed a course of IV vitamin C and weekly testosterone injections after blood testing revealed low levels of the androgen. In addition, under this doctor's direction, Patient G underwent extensive allergy testing, all of which proved negative. Patient G continued under the care of this physician for approximately 5 months before stopping the aggressive treatment when he felt no improvement.

Throughout the early part of 2010, Patient G continued his downward spiral, developing new onset paresthesias in his feet, worsening muscle weakness and pain, ongoing terrible insomnia, and debilitating persistent exhaustion. Finally, during the latter part of 2010, he consulted with yet another "difficult case" internist, hoping this physician might have a solution to his situation. Because of the patient's family history of diabetes, this physician ordered a hemoglobin A_{1c} (HbA_{1c}). This time around, testing revealed a blood sugar close to 500 mg/dL associated with a very high HbA_{1c} near 10%. Oddly, all prior blood sugars had been normal.

Because of the very high blood sugars, Patient G was hospitalized for 2 days with the goal of aggressive supervised insulin treatment of his apparent diabetes along with diabetic teaching, but when discharged his blood sugars remained unstable. At that point, he began experiencing polydipsia, polyphagia, and polyuria. He said that he was thirsty all of the time without ever having a break.

Patient G believed the diabetic teaching given to him in the hospital for self-management of his condition, including the dietary instructions, to be inadequate. Once home, he continued the recommended insulin schedule and tried to incorporate the prescribed eating plan into his life, but nonetheless he could not regulate his sugars properly. He simply did not know how to administer the insulin because the protocol given him seemed unduly complicated, nor was he consistent with the recommended diet. Apparently his doctors did not insist on close medical supervision.

After his hospitalization, Patient G continued experiencing "terrible polyuria and polydipsia" as well as new onset mood swings; at times his temper would go out of control, a new experience for him and his family because he was normally quite mild mannered. During that period, the burning and paresthesias in his feet worsened considerably, particularly if he stood for any length of time.

By the end of 2010, his condition was no better despite the insulin and dietary treatment. Then in January 2011, Patient G developed a severe flu-like illness with fevers, chills, and sweats, so severe that he could barely get out of bed. His throat hurt so badly that he only could consume fluids; at one point, his breathing became labored and he developed new-onset severe midabdominal pain.

In late February 2011, after recovering from his acute flu symptoms, he remained so weak that he could barely walk, and at one point he passed out when attempting to stand up. When he awoke, he felt as if he had "a ton of bricks on his chest." After calling 9-1-1, he was admitted to a local hospital with a body temperature of less than 90°F, in what turned out to be diabetic ketoacidosis with respiratory failure, pneumonia, metabolic acidosis, as well as acute pancreatitis secondary to diabetic ketoacidosis and acute renal failure with secondary acute tubal necrosis from the diabetic ketoacidosis. He was diagnosed as well with mastoiditis and uncorrected hypothyroidism, and he began a 13-treatment course of emergency dialysis for his renal failure. Comorbidly, he developed *Clostridium difficile* pseudomembranous colitis as a result of antibiotic treatment for his pneumonia.

After a difficult 2-week hospitalization, Patient G continued the dialysis as an outpatient. This time around, the endocrinologist (with a history of diabetes himself) assigned to his case prescribed insulin lispro, 4 units 3 times per day, with meals and insulin glargine 50 units at night, and he insisted on close monitoring of his condition. Patient G was also placed on a variety of supplements for his kidney failure including calcium acetate, magnesium oxide, and vitamin B complex. He underwent a course of oral metronidazole for the *Clostridium*, and he was prescribed furosemide 40 mg per day, escitalopram 10 mg per day, levothyroxine 100 µg per day, and a probiotic. With careful management, Patient G's diabetes seemed finally under, if not ideal, at least better control.

In early June 2011, 2 weeks before his first consultation with this medical doctor (MD), Patient G consulted an ophthalmologist who found, fortunately, no damage to his eyes.

Our evaluation of all new patients, whatever their underlying problem might be, involves 2 lengthy sessions. The first is the intake history and physical, which usually takes 2 hours because the majority of our patients tend to present to us, as in this case, with complicated medical histories. During the second session, again usually lasting 2 hours, we review the recommended nutritional protocol in some depth.

At the time of our first meeting together, Patient G appeared very fatigued, worn out, and pale. He did not smile once through the 2-hour session and at times talking seemed to be an effort. He still was out of work, but he did explain that in recent weeks, with close medical management, better dietary compliance, and a regular program of insulin lispro and insulin glargine, his blood sugars had been fairly well regulated and some of his symptoms had lessened in severity. He reported that the hair on his arms and legs had begun regrowing; his gums showed some improvement, but he still required zolpidem for persistent severe insomnia and the paresthesias in his feet had actually worsened. He described burning in his feet so intense he could not stand for any length of time and he experienced persistent odd "electrical-shock" type symptoms in various places in his body.

His endocrinologist had arranged teaching for intensive foot care, which Patient G followed to the letter, washing his feet 3 to 4 times daily. His sexual function, though improved, remained problematic, perhaps, as he said, 20% of his former self. He had some time earlier discontinued the testosterone prescribed by one of his alternative doctors because he felt it did nothing. He still could not exercise because of his persistent weakness and fatigue as well as the paresthesias in his feet that made activity such as running or walking impossible. He described chronic loose, watery stool associated with some urgency maybe twice per day; some lower back pain; and muscle cramping at night in his calves.

He reported occasional chills but no sweats, and bouts of nausea, which he related to low blood sugars. Because Patient G could go from hyperglycemia to hypoglycemia very quickly, his endocrinologist had advised him not to use the insulin lispro if he had not eaten.

His most recent blood work from early May 2011 showed an HbA_{1c} high at 7.8%; a normal TSH at 4.01 mIU/L; a high glucose at 133 mg/dL; and normal blood urea nitrogen (BUN), creatinine, electrolytes, and liver function. A complete blood count (CBC) from March indicated a low hemoglobin at 9.8 g/dL with a hematocrit at 29.4%. A recent CT scan of his brain had revealed some cerebral edema.

Under past medical history, the following problems were listed:

1. Insulin-dependent diabetes.
2. Acute renal failure requiring 13 treatments of dialysis in February/March 2011.
3. Hypothyroidism.
4. Diabetic ketoacidosis.
5. Pancreatitis.
6. Pseudomembranous colitis.
7. Periodontal disease.
8. Occasional migraines.
9. Hypoglycemia with syncope if he does not eat. Two MRI scans have been negative.
10. Pneumonia when he was admitted into the hospital in February 2011.
11. Chronic diarrhea.
12. Borderline hypertension.

At the time of his first visit with this MD, Patient G's medications included hydrochlorothiazide 20 mg per day, duloxetine 30 mg per day for muscle pain, insulin lispro 4 units 3 times per day with meals, and insulin glargine 50 units at bedtime. He remained on levothyroxine 100 µg each morning.

On physical examination, Patient G's blood pressure was mildly elevated at 136/100 mm Hg. Other than lack of hair on his extremities, he appeared otherwise normal.

Notably, despite a family history of diabetes, this patient's dysglycemia is likely of traumatic/mechanical etiology related to his injury in 2007 that most likely had damaged his pancreas significantly, setting the stage for his subsequent decline.

During the second session, we reviewed at length the proposed treatment plan. In general, our therapy can be broken down into 3 basic components: individualized diet, individualized supplement protocols, and detoxification routines such as coffee enemas. Unlike many alternative practitioners, we do not prescribe one diet for everyone, but we recommend very detailed and individualized eating plans based on our assessment of each patient's underlying metabolism. Our prescribed diets can range from largely raw food plant-based—though we never recommend a purely vegetarian diet—to an Atkins'-type diet emphasizing multiple courses of fatty red meat daily, with all manner of diets in between. Similarly, we prescribe a variety of supplements, including vitamins, minerals, trace metals, enzymes and glandular products (made for us in New Zealand), the doses, forms, and proportions varying, again depending on our assessment of the patient's metabolic needs. For all patients, whatever their problem and whatever their prescribed diet and supplement regimen, we require the coffee enemas and other procedures such as a liver flush, colon cleanses, juice fasts, and various baths.

NUTRITION AND THE AUTONOMIC NERVOUS SYSTEM

We base our dietary and supplemental prescriptions on the state of the patient's autonomic nervous system (ANS), whose 2 branches, the sympathetic and parasympathetic, regulate all or most all metabolism including respiration, cardiovascular function, digestion, endocrine activity, and immunity. Certain patients we believe have a genetically determined tonically active, even hyperactive, sympathetic nervous system (SNS) and a correspondingly weak parasympathetic nervous system (PNS). In these patients, all those tissues, organs, and glands normally stimulated by the SNS such as the organs of respiration, cardiovascular function, and endocrine secretion, tend to be highly developed and overly efficient, whereas those tissues, organs, and glands normally stimulated by the weak parasympathetic system, such as all the digestive organs including the liver and pancreas as well as the immune system, tend to be weak and inefficient. These patients, we find, respond best to a plant-based diet, though the exact composition varies depending on the degree of what we call "sympathetic dominance."

Other patients, we find, possess an overly strong, genetically determined parasympathetic system, and a correspondingly weak sympathetic system. In these patients those tissues, organs, and glands normally stimulated by the PNS, particularly those of digestion and immunity, tend to be highly active, even overactive, whereas those tissues, organs, and glands normally stimulated by their weak SNS, such as the lungs and heart, tend to be inefficient.

The third category demonstrates a balanced autonomic system, with both branches equally developed and equally efficient. In this group all the various physiological systems and their associated tissues, organs, and glands, work equally effectively.

Such a construct is of more than only esoteric interest, and in our model it helps explain the origins of much disease while providing insight into beneficial treatment approaches. Fundamentally, we perceive that much if not most illness including malignancy develops either because of autonomic imbalance, or in the case of "balanced metabolizers," combined inefficiency in both the SNS and PNS divisions.

The concept that autonomic imbalance or autonomic inefficiency underscores much disease did not originate in our office, but to the contrary has a long and well-researched history going back nearly 100 years. Francis Pottenger Sr, MD, son of the famed Pottenger medical family with now 4 generations of American physicians to its roster, described the critical role of autonomic activity, autonomic imbalance, and autonomic inefficiency in his classic text *Symptoms of Visceral Disease* with 6 editions beginning in 1922 and the last dating to 1944.[7]

The great University of Minnesota physician and neuroscientist, Ernst Gellhorn, MD, PhD, with more than 400 papers and 8 books to his credit, spent decades investigating the role of autonomic imbalance and inefficiency as the root cause of much human illness.[8] Succeeding Pottenger and Gellhorn, the more unconventional alternative practitioner, the dentist William Donald Kelley, combined the work of these 2 scientists into a complex nutritional therapy based on autonomic dysfunction.[9]

It was Kelley who first proposed that the typical solid epithelial tumors—that is tumors of the breast, lung, pancreas, colon, liver, uterus, ovaries, and prostate—tend to develop in those with a strong sympathetic system and weak parasympathetic system. In contrast, immune malignancies such as leukemia, lymphoma and multiple myeloma, and the embryologically related connective tissue cancers such as the sarcomas, occur in those with a strong PNS and a weak SNS. Balanced autonomic metabolizers tend to avoid cancer, though they can experience other illnesses and syndromes such as chronic fatigue if both branches weaken.

In these models of Pottenger, Gellhorn, and Kelley, restoration of health, whatever the underlying problems, requires bringing an out-of-balance autonomic system into balance and homeostatic equilibrium, or in the case of balanced metabolizers, improving efficiency and synergy in both autonomic divisions.

Both Pottenger and Gellhorn, independently of each other, had discovered that certain nutrients, particularly minerals such as calcium, magnesium, and potassium—whatever else they might do in the body—have an enormous influence on autonomic firing. For example, Pottenger discovered that calcium stimulates the SNS, magnesium blocks sympathetic firing at the ganglion, and potassium stimulates the PNS in central nuclei. By judicious use of nutrients such as these, Pottenger, in his clinical work with patients, could successfully bring an out-of-balance autonomic system into balance or improve the efficiency of each. Gellhorn, in his research, further confirmed the profound influence of various nutrients on autonomic function, showing again, as had Pottenger, that by their precise use autonomic balance and autonomic efficiency would improve, with often startling positive results in his clinic patients.

Though these pioneering researchers concentrated on certain nutrients, it was Kelley who would more thoroughly investigate the precise effect of foods and the various individual nutrients—the vitamins, minerals, trace elements, fatty acids, etc—on autonomic activity. And in his dietary and supplement prescriptions, Dr Kelley always sought to bring an out-of-balance ANS into efficient equilibrium— or with his "balanced metabolizers," strengthen both branches equally.

Dr Kelley believed that his "sympathetic dominant" patients, whatever the underlying problem, required for improvement a plant-based diet that included a wide variety of fruits, vegetables, nuts, seeds, and organic whole-grain products but limited animal protein, eggs, yogurt, and cheese, with some additional food from animal sources depending on the extent of sympathetic activity; the stronger the SNS, the fewer animal products he would allow.

As more conventional nutritional scientists know, vegetables and fruits have an alkaline ash, and an alkaline extracellular fluid environment tends to suppress sympathetic, while increasing parasympathetic, firing. Further, fruits and vegetables provide significant amounts of the minerals magnesium and potassium, which as Pottenger had shown, respectively suppress sympathetic tone while increasing that of the parasympathetic nerves.

Red meat and to some extent poultry provide certain nutrients in relatively high amounts such as phosphates, sulfates, the amino acids phenylalanine, tyrosine, aspartic acid, glutamic acid, and saturated fats, all of which, via unique pathways, stimulate the SNS while suppressing the PNS. The phosphates and sulfates, for example, convert in the body into phosphoric and sulfuric acid, acidifying extracellular fluids and in turn activating the SNS while suppressing the PNS—a scenario what would be counterproductive for a sympathetic dominant metabolizer. Phenylalanine and tyrosine, which serve as the precursors to the sympathetic neurotransmitters norepinephrine and epinephrine, similarly have a SNS stimulating effect. So in a sympathetic dominant patient we restrict these animal foods, the amounts allowed again depending on the degree of sympathetic dominance. In an extremely strong sympathetic dominant we forbid all red meat and poultry; for a patient only slightly on the side of sympathetic dominance we might allow small amounts of both weekly.

In summary, a largely plant-based diet specifically suppresses the sympathetic division while activating the parasympathetics.

In his day, Dr Kelley prescribed—and we recommend today—precise forms, doses, and proportions of the various vitamins, minerals, trace elements, at times herbs and often glandular products from New Zealand animals, again designed, like diet, to bring about autonomic balance and efficiency. ANS balance is always our main concern in any of our dietary or supplement prescriptions. Of course all the various individual nutrients have multiple metabolic roles—magnesium for example serves as a cofactor in more than 300 reactions—but our concern is always their effect on the autonomic system.

Specifically, Kelley found and we find that β-carotene, the B vitamins thiamine, riboflavin, niacin, pyridoxine, folic acid, and vitamins C and D either suppress the SNS or stimulate the PNS. Certain minerals and trace elements including magnesium, potassium, manganese, and chromium, have a similar SNS-inhibiting, PNS-activating action as does the plant-based omega-3 essential fatty acid, α-linolenic acid.

For the parasympathetic-dominant patients, Kelley prescribed—and we prescribe today—a diet high in animal fats and protein, sometimes red meat twice daily, which with its specific complement of nutrients such as the phosphates sulfates, phenylalanine, tyrosine, aspartic acid, glutamic acid, and saturated fatty acids, will stimulate the weak SNS and suppress the strong PNS, helping to bring the out-of-balance ANS in the parasympathetic dominant patients into more efficient equilibrium. With their acid-forming, sympathetic stimulating activity, meat and poultry represent ideal foods for this group of patients—again the frequency and amounts varying according to the degree of parasympathetic dominance; the more parasympathetic a patient, the more fatty red meat we prescribe.

Parasympathetic dominant patients do well with certain vegetables, particularly root vegetables and those in the cruciferous family, which we find to be not particularly alkalinizing, but the diets limit or forbid leafy greens which, because of their high magnesium content, will suppress the SNS. For our parasympathetic patients we allow varying amounts of whole organic grains, again the amount depending on the extent of PNS dominance; the more parasympathetic a patient, the fewer servings of grains we allow. The diet does permit beans but limited or no fruit. Fruit, with its alkaline ash, its high content of potassium and other SNS-suppressing nutrients, would be counterproductive for this group. For a patient with an extremely strong PNS, we restrict fruits and grains to the point that, at times, we allow none at all.

Parasympathetics do best with certain nutrients, specifically preformed vitamin A; certain B vitamins including B_{12}, choline, inositol, PABA, and pantothenic acid: and the calcium salts of vitamin C and vitamin E. Appropriate minerals include large doses of calcium, which we find stimulates strongly the SNS (but minimal amounts of magnesium and potassium); the trace minerals selenium and zinc; and the animal-derived omega-3 fatty acids, eicosapentaenoic acid (EPA) and docosahexaenoic acid (DHA), which we find best suited to their metabolic needs.

Balanced metabolizers do best with a diet and supplement regimen that provides all the food classes and nutrients but in moderate doses that will effectively stimulate and support both autonomic branches equally, helping to promote and maintain efficient autonomic function and autonomic balance. For this group the diet allows all the various fruits, vegetables, nuts, seeds, whole grains, eggs daily, organic raw milk and raw cheese, fish 2 to 3 times weekly, poultry 2 to 3 times weekly, and red meat 2 to 4 times weekly. In terms of supplements, for these patients, we prescribe all the various vitamins, minerals, trace elements, and essential fatty acids (from both plant and animal sources) but in moderate doses so as not to excessively stimulate or suppress either autonomic branch.

OUR APPROACH TO DIABETES

Kelly recognized, as do endocrinologists, 2 forms of diabetes: an insulin-deficient type and an insulin-excess variety—what we would today call *insulin resistance*. But his approach, as does ours today, differed considerably from conventional wisdom, always focusing as he did on autonomic activity and imbalance as the underlying culprit needing to be addressed.

If for a moment we think of diabetes in autonomic terms, indeed when the sympathetic system fires, it does suppress both the exocrine and endocrine pancreas while stimulating gluconeogenesis, leading to a combination of diminished insulin secretion, increased glucose production and, consequently, chronically low blood insulin, elevated blood sugars, and elevated HbA_{1c}. In Kelley's model, a sympathetic dominant individual who might follow the typical American eating plan including 150 pounds of white sugar a year, and an additional regular intake of refined and processed grains and food, will end up with an insulin deficient form of the disease prompted by carbohydrate excess in the absence of β-cell reserve.

When the parasympathetic nerves fire, they increase both the synthesis and the release of insulin, while stimulating the storage of glucose either as glycogen or in adipocytes as triglycerides. In these patients, an intake of white sugar and refined grains leads first to reactive hypoglycemia due to the hyperinsulinemia, followed by classic insulin resistance. In this situation, the excessive blood levels of insulin provoke insensitivity in the insulin receptor of target cells, which when functionally normal will activate the downstream glucose membrane receptor so the sugar can enter cells to be used for energy,

In the world of mainstream diabetic thinking, physicians believe the "insulin-dependent, type 1" or childhood diabetes results from alleged autoimmune attack on and destruction of the insulin-secreting β cells of the pancreas often occurring at quite young ages. Kelley believed this type of insulin-deficient diabetes could occur in adults as well as in children, and even in the group of child patients, the real culprit remained an excessively active SNS, perhaps beginning during fetal growth and development. The traditional type 2 form, more easily regulated by diet, would be consistent with Stanford researcher Dr Gerald Reavens concept of insulin resistance, persistent insulin excess in response to a high intake of poor quality refined carbohydrates, leading eventually to receptor insensitivity and the paradoxical situation of high blood insulin and high blood glucose.

In the case of Patient G, the initial evaluation of his autonomic status indicated that he fell moderately into sympathetic dominance but not extremely so. For him, I prescribed what we call the "Balanced Vegetarian Metabolizer Diet" designed for those patients who are essentially balanced in terms of autonomic efficiency but leaning toward sympathetic dominance.

CASE REPORT CONTINUED: PATIENT G'S SPECIFIC DIET

As a first principle for all our patients, whatever their autonomic state and whatever their prescribed diet, we strongly advise that their food be organic, as clean as possible, and always non-GMO. Studies going back to the great English agronomist Sir Albert Howard repeatedly have demonstrated the superior nutritional value of "organically" raised foods and livestock. Such agricultural practices provide additional benefit to the soil and the various soil organisms such as earthworms and the microorganisms of the soil; this microbiome forms the foundation of all agriculture and is susceptible to damage from pesticides and herbicides. To make matters worse, pesticides, at least most of them, act as neurotoxins, which we believe should be avoided at all costs.

I recommended for Patient G that approximately 50% of his food be consumed in the raw, uncooked state, whereas 50% should be cooked. Researchers such as the late Edward Howell proposed that raw food contains all the vitamins, minerals, and trace elements in a completely undamaged and usually more accessible form than does cooked food.[10] In addition, Howell pointed out that every cell, whether from a plant or animal, contains hundreds of different enzymes as part of the cell's normal metabolic machinery. These enzymes, Howell maintained, based on his clinical and laboratory studies, could be absorbed like a vitamin or mineral to assist in various metabolic reactions and help in the repair and rebuilding of damaged tissue.

However, these "food enzymes," as Howell called them, denature and deactivate above 117°F (47°C) so even mild cooking will render them useless as beneficial nutrients. Because of this finding, Howell became a great proponent of raw food therapeutic diets, projecting him into the role of grandfather of the current "raw foods" movement.

Though Kelley acknowledged the benefits of raw food, he also learned, through his extensive clinical experience, that some patients did best with mostly cooked food. For those who might have been ravaged by cancer and aggressive conventional treatments such as chemotherapy and radiation, Kelley found their digestion to be so inefficient they could not tolerate an excess of raw food. Though cooking does neutralize certain nutrients such as folic acid and vitamin C, make certain minerals like calcium less available, and inactive the "food enzymes," the process does break down cell walls and membranes in plant and animal food products respectively, in a sense "predigesting" the food, thereby making it more easily assimilated. To make up for any nutrient loss in the cooking process, Kelley would always prescribe—as we do today—large doses of accessory nutrients and an enzyme product developed by Dr Howell himself. In any event, we find balanced metabolizers particularly, such as Patient G, do best with a diet equally proportioned between cooked and raw.

In terms of specific food types, the diet prescribed Patient G allowed all the different vegetables, encouraging the intake of at least 3 to 4 servings per day with a mix of both cooked vegetables and raw vegetables in salads and freshly made juice, with no limit whatsoever on serving size or frequency. The diet did recommend frequent servings from the cruciferous family which have an anticancer effect, as well as dark leafy greens, which provide a significant amount of magnesium and a sympathetic-suppressing effect, ideally suited for a patient such as Patient G who fell, if only mildly, on the sympathetic dominant side.

The prescribed diet also included a glass of freshly made carrot juice daily, which we find provides a host of useful nutrients and enzymes. We find that, in a patient such as this with a strong SNS and what we consider an "insulin-deficient" form of diabetes, the sugar content in a single glass of carrot juice does not affect the blood glucose to any great extent; the benefit, we believe, far exceeds any small risk.

Despite current recommendations in some camps that diabetics of any ilk should avoid all fruit, Patient G was allowed as much *whole* as desired, but restricted fruit juice and dried fruit whose concentrated sugar content would be initially excessive. In addition, balanced vegetarian metabolizers diagnosed with diabetes tolerate grains, even gluten, well, as long as they consume non-GMO organic forms, preferably sprouted such as the Ezekiel line of breads and grain products. Such grain foods tend to be not only more nutritious as the sprouting process increases the enzyme content but also less allergenic. In any event, we do not find that these foods significantly and negatively affect blood glucose levels in this specific group of patients as long as they stick to the organic, non-GMO, preferably sprouted forms.

The diet also allowed as much, or as little, of the nuts, seeds, and bean categories as Patient G might wish to consume, though again emphasizing organic non-GMO varieties in all cases, while forbidding peanuts and soy. Peanuts, technically a legume, can grow the *Aspergillus* mold, which produces the liver toxin, aflatoxin. Though there remains ongoing debate about the potential problem this is in US-grown peanuts, we err on the side of caution. And we forbid for all our patients soy products, even though they are widely promoted as a "health food," for 2 reasons. First, a regular intake of soy will, in time, block thyroid function, eventually leading to hypothyroidism. Second, soy contains the protein Bowman-Birk inhibitor, named for the scientists who isolated it, that interferes with the action of trypsin, the main pancreatic proteolytic enzyme so important in our anticancer programs.

Though Patient G tended toward the sympathetic dominant side, because he fell close to balance, I did allow in his diet a fair amount of animal protein, including 2 organic eggs daily, cooked anyway he preferred, and raw milk to drink as well as raw milk cheese, yogurt, and butter. Evidence dating back to the famed cat studies of Francis Pottenger, Jr, son of the previously mentioned neuroscientist Pottenger, that he conducted for 10 years beginning in 1932 rather forcefully documented the dangers of cooked milk and as opposed to the health-promoting qualities of raw milk. Today, the current industry practice of heating milk to 230°F (110°C) and separating, recombining, and homogenizing the fat and watery liquid effectively destroys all the important enzymes and many other nutrients as well. Kurt Oster of Bridgeport, Connecticut, long argued that the cherished process of homogenization changed the milk into an atherosclerosis-provoking food.[11] Of course, most states forbid the retail sale of raw milk, but even in those locales, patients can often obtain raw milk from local farmers or buyer's groups.

I also recommended 2 to 3 servings of seafood weekly. We fully recognize the increasing problems of pollution of our major and minor waterways, which affects the quality of the fish living in these waters. But there are still areas, as in the Alaskan inlets and waterways and in the North Atlantic, that provide clean fish, or as clean as one can find in this day and age. For all our patients, we do forbid the large predatory fish such as tuna and swordfish that accumulate mercury with time, as well as farm raised fish, much of which now comes from South Asia and China, where there are lax environmental regulations and questionable growing methods.

The diet allowed 2 to 3 servings of organically-raised poultry per week and 2 to 4 servings of grass-fed fatty red meat. For the fish, poultry and red meat, I prescribed a specific frequency per week, but in all cases left the actual serving size up the patient. I learned a long time ago from Dr Kelley that a patient's brain will be a far more accurate guide in determining appropriate serving sizes than some preconceived arbitrary rule.

I thought, based on my experience, that the weekly servings of acid-forming, sympathetic stimulating red meat were necessary in this case to help achieve balance in the autonomic branches. A diet too heavy in fruits and vegetables in a patient such as this, and lacking sufficient animal foods, would in our experience push him too strongly into parasympathetic dominance, excessive production of insulin, and, down the road, an insulin-resistance type of diabetes. We find that the recommended servings of animal products in a slightly sympathetic dominant patient keep the pendulum from swinging too far into the parasympathetic realm, preventing a whole other set of problems.

The supplement protocol I designed for Patient G totaled 26 capsules with breakfast and dinner, and 37 with lunch. His program included what we call the "Moderate Vegetarian Multi Min" providing those minerals and trace metals such as magnesium, potassium, chromium, and manganese that we find suppress the SNS and activate the PNS. A separate supplement, the "Moderate Vegetarian Multi Vit," as it is called, contains those vitamins that we find similarly suppress the SNS while increasing parasympathetic tone, such as β-carotene, the B vitamins thiamine, riboflavin, niacin, folate, and pyridoxine, and vitamin C and vitamin D. In addition, I included a Glucose Tolerance Factor supplement consisting of chromium and associated nutrients that have been documented to help regulate sugar metabolism and which we find particularly useful for our sympathetic dominant patients. For added benefit, Patient Gs program included the antioxidant α-lipoic acid and the amino acid *N*-acetylcysteine, a duo that together increases levels of glutathione in the body and, like chromium, assists in glucose regulation. For all patients, we also recommend a probiotic, most commonly "Vital 10" from Klaire Labs. In addition, in Patient G's particular case I also added a capsule of *Saccharomyces boulardii*, a specific bacterium found useful in those patients recovering from *Clostridium difficile* infection.

Patient G's supplement protocol provided a number of "glandular" products in capsule form including adrenal medulla, hypothalamus, liver, and orchic (testicle), derived from animals and made for us in New Zealand by exacting technology. Such supplements, we believe, provide certain growth factors that target like tissues, enhancing repair and regeneration of damaged cells. With each meal, I also prescribed 6 capsules of our pancreas enzyme product, which contains the various digestive enzymes but also homeopathic doses of insulin. In the whole pancreas glandular concentrate, we find that the insulin seems to be absorbed active into the blood stream, in contrast to purified preparations of insulin, which denature in the stomach when taken orally. In the 1920s, before the wide availability of manufactured insulin, physicians at times would prescribe whole pancreas supplements that seemed to keep the disease in check.

As part of the third component of Patient G's treatment regimen, the detoxification routines I prescribed included daily coffee enemas, which we believe are as important to treatment success as the recommended diet and supplement protocols. We find that as a patient's body repairs and rebuilds, regardless of the underlying problem, large amounts of toxic debris will be released from stored sites within the various cells. These wastes include sequestered toxic chemicals from environmental sources such as heavy metals, pesticides, hydrocarbons, etc, that sit in the cells waiting to cause genetic and cytoplasmic damage. In addition, wastes from normal cellular metabolism can also accumulate, adding to the deleterious load. In our program, with all the good nutrition provided, it appears that the various cells get the signal to begin molecular "house cleaning," gradually dumping the stored toxins and metabolic wastes into the blood stream for eventual processing and excretion primarily through the liver and secondarily through the kidneys. Because of inefficiency in our natural detoxification systems due to chronic overexposure to environmental chemicals and processed food, we find adjunctive "detoxification" a critical component of the therapy.

The mainstay of the detoxification routines remains for all patients the daily coffee enemas, which have long been belittled by the conventional medical world. However, I have found few physicians aware that esteemed medical texts, including the *Merck Manual*, and many conventional nursing texts, recommended coffee enemas as a treatment modality for decades during the 20th century. In addition, there exist dozens of papers from the academic peer-reviewed literature beginning in the 1920s documenting the effective use of coffee and other forms of enemas in syndromes as variable as septic shock and arthritis to bipolar illness. One memorable paper from the *New England Journal of Medicine* in 1932[12] reports the successful treatment of hospitalized psychiatric patients with a variety of "colonic irrigations."

We believe that the coffee enemas, through activation of a parasympathetic reflex, stimulate both phase 1 and phase 2 detoxification systems in the liver, whose efficient function is so important in the treatment of just about any disease. For Patient G, I also prescribed other procedures such as a liver flush and a colon cleanse, to be alternated on a monthly basis. For most of our patients we usually recommend any of a number of juice fasts, but in this patient's case, because of the unstable blood sugar picture, I thought any juice fast would be too strenuous early on in the treatment process.

Because of G's terrible chronic insomnia, I prescribed the "blue light blocking glasses" available from Photonic Developments (Walton Hills, OH, USA). This intervention is based on the discovery that all light, whether natural sunlight in origin or artificial from light bulbs, TV screens, computers, smart phone screens, etc, contains a blue wave length, which is most commonly invisible to the eye. This particular light wavelength stimulates the alert centers in the brain as a survival benefit to keep us awake and aware in daylight. Like any daytime creature, our circadian rhythms dictate that we should be alert during daylight, and sleepy at night, when under natural conditions with the setting of the sun, the stimulating blue light wavelength disappears. But we creative humans with our synthetic lights and electronic devices expose our brain to an ongoing barrage of blue wavelength light that keeps us in an "unnatural" state of vigilance in preparation for activity, even well into late night. An outcome of disrupted sleep cycles and chronic insomnia often follows.

My patient's research group designed eyeglasses, akin to sunglasses, with a rose colored lens that blocks specifically and only the blue light, in effect tricking the brain into thinking it is pitch dark even when surrounded by light. With the activating centers of the brain turned off, we can fall asleep normally, even if living in a light-rich environment and continuing our activities, such as TV-watching or computer work—as long as we wear the blue light blocking glasses. In clinical trials, the glasses worked well, bringing on sleepiness quickly, often in the most hardened of insomniacs. For years, I have been prescribing the blue light blocking glasses for patients with a history of insomnia, usually with satisfying outcomes.

During the second 2-hour session with Patient G and his wife, I reviewed in great detail the various aspects of the prescribed protocol. By the end of that meeting, when he expressed his gratitude that I was willing to take him on as a patient, I suspected he would be compliant with all aspects of the treatment. As we parted, after the second part of the consultation, the patient expressed understanding of the treatment and was encouraged to call with any questions he might have, also suggesting that, because he lived fairly close to New York City, he return for an office visit in 3 months.

PATIENT G'S PROGRESS ON THE THERAPY

For all my patients, wherever they may live, we require that they return for an extended re-evaluation every 6 months. More-local patients, such as Patient G, I like to monitor initially closely, usually every 3 months, but after our initial 2 sessions together, Patient G disappeared for an extended time. In the months that followed our initial sessions together, not once did he call with a question. There was no contact until he sent a Christmas card in late December 2011, adding to the printed message, "Thank you for getting my life back in order." I assumed he must be doing well, but I would not hear from him again until he came in for an appointment in mid-June 2012—a year after he had first consulted with me.

At that time, he walked in, again with his wife, looking like a completely different individual from a year earlier. First of all, he was smiling, in stark contrast to his pained visage during our first sessions and he had what might be best described as a "glow" of good health. He expressed gratefully that the "the program has changed my life." He apologized for not coming in sooner as I had recommended, but he had been out of work until recently, so money had been tight. But he was pleased to inform me that now he had a good job he enjoyed and his newfound excellent energy, stamina, and concentration, which he attributed to the nutritional regimen that allowed him now to work long hours under stress without any difficulty.

During the previous 12 months, Patient G had been vigilantly compliant with all aspects of the prescribed nutritional program, including the diet, supplements, and detoxification routines. When we talked about his apparent good compliance, he had a very simple answer—I had told him what he needed to do, and he just went ahead and did it all, without complaint or need for constant support from me.

My note from the day sums up his current situation:

> He said that he is doing so much better. He said that when he walked in here he could barely function. He said that his functionality is extraordinary. He has been extremely compliant with all aspects of the problem. … He does the whole program.

> In addition, he is on insulin lispro, which he takes three times a day. He varies the dose according to his blood sugars. He is also on insulin glargine and down to about 25 to 30 units at bedtime. He was on 50 units when he first came in. … He is off the duloxetine.

> He basically emphasized that the program has changed his life …

> He is enjoying his work and working long hours.

> He said that when he came in here one year ago he could not exercise at all. He is exercising regularly. He is going to the gym. He is lifting weights …

> He said that he is enjoying his life. He is enjoying his children. He said that it is just wonderful to be alive. He said that the program has made "an unbelievable difference" in his life. His energy is substantially improved. He is able to enjoy life, go out, and be with his children. He said that he could not do that one year ago when he came in here because he was so weak, exhausted, tired, and sick. He is using much less insulin. His endocrinologist, who knows he sees me, is extremely happy with how he is doing …

> He said that for so long he was not exercising but he is now feeling so good that he can exercise. He does not need the duloxetine anymore for the muscle pain.

> The blue light blocking glasses helped enormously with his sleep. He said that they were "miraculous." He is sleeping soundly and sleeping well.

> His energy is "unbelievable." Stamina is "great." Concentration is "very good."

> His kidneys are fine. They did kidney function tests three months ago that were perfect, as if he had never been sick. Nephrologist has discharged him as he does not need to see him anymore.

In addition, Patient G's periodontal disease had completely resolved, he had not experienced any further episodes of pancreatitis, his gastrointestinal function was now completely normal, and he rarely felt hypoglycemic.

Based on my testing, my experience, and his excellent clinical situation, no changes were made to his prescribed diet and only very minor alterations in his supplement protocol. He was to continue the detoxification routines as before.

Subsequently, Patient G continued as a "low maintenance" patient. For the next 6 months, he did not call once with a question or problem, and I would not hear from him again until he and his wife returned to my office in mid-December 2012, some 18 months after his first beginning treatment with me.

Again he looked well, reported feeling well and remained very compliant with his nutritional regimen. My note from the session recorded his situation at the time:

> He looks great. He said that he is feeling great. His job is going well. … He is busy and he is doing well financially. When he first came in here, as he said today, he did not have a job and he said that he could not work. He had lost his job because he could not function …

> He said that he is really doing fine. He continues on the insulin lispro but is adjusting the dose downward. He does not need as much. … He is really exercising quite vigorously …

> He said that his stamina is "fantastic." Energy is "fantastic … " He is sleeping well. He said that the blue light blocking glasses really changed his sleep …

> The only doctor he is seeing at this point is his endocrinologist. … He has not done blood work so I suggested that we need to do that. He agreed. He said that he just does not want to see any other doctors other than me. His endocrinologist … is just monitoring his blood sugars. His hemoglobin A_{1C} last time was 12 …

Although I had given him an order for extensive blood testing at our December 2012 meeting, he would not get the test done until late June 2013, in preparation for his upcoming re-evaluation scheduled for the second week of July 2013—now 2 years since he had begun treatment with me. At that time, his blood sugars seemed less controlled, coming in at 328 mg/dL with a significantly elevated HbA_{1c} at 14% (normal 4.8%-5.6%). His TSH was also elevated at 6.24 mIU/L (normal 0.45-4.50 mIU/L). Though he had remained on levothyroxine, clearly he needed more thyroid replacement, or a different form of medication.

Upon follow-up, he looked well, seemed—as before—completely compliant with the therapy, and expressed—once again—his heartfelt gratitude for the treatment. He informed me that he felt so well he had taken on a second full-time job because of his family's financial needs but felt terrific despite the added workload. I thought it a sign of great progress that he could manage 2 stressful jobs successfully, because when he had first consulted me, he could not work at all. He also explained that he, his wife, and his children had just returned from a 2-week vacation out west, including a trip to the Grand Canyon, which he had enjoyed immensely. As my note recorded, "He said that it was really very relaxing and he really enjoyed it."

Regarding blood sugar instability, he reported that his daily blood sugar monitoring generally indicated a level no higher than 200 mg/dL. Based on clinical experience, it was suspected that the problem might be stress brought on by his second job. Compliance with diet and the prescribed supplements did not seem to be an issue, because he appeared to be as dedicated as ever to the treatment. But he did acknowledge recent significant additional stresses in his life.

As my note from the visit reported:

> He has been under a lot of stress, and I could tell from the metabolic report. He took a second job. He is a salesman for medical products. ... They are completely different products so he is able to do that without a conflict of interest. He is working anywhere from 10 to 16 hours a day. His territory. ... goes from Washington D.C. up to New Hampshire.

> He said that he just needed the extra money with his three kids. ... It is a lot of stress. He said that the miracle is that he is able to do it. He is able to work 12 to 16-hour days. He has good energy, stamina, and endurance. We talked at length about the fact that this is really too much considering where he came from as he was really burnt out when he first walked into my office. He said that he really feels "great."

> His blood sugars at home range around 200 mg/dl.

> He has been working out three to five times a week. He said that the miracle is that when he first came in [sic] could not work at all. ... His energy, he said, is great. Stamina is "great." Concentration is good. He is sleeping great. He said that the blue light blocking glasses really made a difference.

Because of his high TSH, I increased his kelp supplement, a good source of iodine, and the thyroid glandular we use with patients experiencing hypothyroidism. Because he was due to see his endocrinologist in 2 weeks, adjustments to levothyroxine dose were deferred.

It was not surprising, based on increased work stress, that his blood sugar picture had become a problem; as patients improve on our therapy and start feeling truly well after long periods of severe ill health, they may take on more activities and responsibilities than I would normally recommend. Particularly with Patient G's autonomic profile, increased stress was almost guaranteed, at least at this still early point in his therapy with me, to worsen his blood sugars. Stress in any form in a patient such as this with a dominant SNS, whether it be physical, psychological, spiritual, or—as in this case—work-related, turns on the sympathetic system more strongly, turns off the parasympathetic system, and reduces insulin synthesis and secretion.

In preparation for Patient G's next visit with me in mid-January 2014—2.5 years after his first consultation—blood testing indicated some improvement, with his blood sugar down to 280 mg/dL and HbA$_{1c}$ at 12.4%. His TSH had actually worsened to 8.43 mIU/L. Despite these results, when he was examined, he looked well, remained compliant with all aspects of his therapy, and reported that he was "doing great." After seeing me in July 2013, and despite his misgivings, he had consulted again with his endocrinologist who had doubled his levothyroxine dose to 200 μg daily.

Fortunately, he had quit the more demanding of his 2 jobs, the one that required considerable travel, which he did not enjoy, and which he admitted had affected his sense of well-being. Instead, he had taken on another second full-time job, but one that required only local travel and which he found more intellectually stimulating although less stressful. As I wrote in my note, "… he is very happy with his job and felt my advice was really very useful."

He continued his regular strenuous workouts, which he acknowledged did help control his blood sugar levels, enabling him to reduce his insulin dosing still further. He also remarked that through trial and error he realized that when his blood sugar went below 120 mg/dL, he did not feel well at all, observing that a level between 120 and 150 mg/dL seemed most suitable, leaving him feeling most energetic and alert. We do find that our sympathetic dominant patients in general, and our sympathetic diabetic patients in particular, not only tolerate what would be considered higher than normal blood sugars, but, as in this case, feel best with moderately elevated blood glucose and feel terrible with sugars in the so-called optimal range.

My note described his continuing good health: "Overall his energy is excellent. Stamina is good. He gets through the day fine. He is sleeping 'great.' He does not even have to use the blue light blocking glasses anymore as sleep as improved so much. Concentration is good."

After discussing his worsening TSH result, I decided to up his dose of our nonprescription thyroid support supplement, to 2 at breakfast, 2 at dinner, and 1 at lunch.

When I next saw Patient G in mid-July 2014, he had completed 3 years of treatment with me, remained compliant, and continued improving. Again, he reported that the therapy "has changed my life."

Though he had not gone for the blood testing I had requested for the visit, he reported that with increasing vigorous exercise, in the past 6 months his blood sugars had further stabilized, rarely going below 120 or above 150 mg/dL. The levels tended to be highest in the AM, then improved throughout the day. As before, with these levels he seemed to feel clinically the best.

His assessment in comparison to his original set of health problems was as follows:

> He has had no recurrences of any of the diarrhea or pseudo-membranous colitis type symptoms. He said his gut is "fine."

> He has been to his dentist and his gums and teeth are fine.

> He has been to his ophthalmologist and there is no damage at all to his retina. His ophthalmologist is very pleased.

> He has very rare hypoglycemic symptoms. He knows how to manage them well …

> He has also had no further recurrences of any of his pancreatitis type symptoms. … He is really doing very well.

> He has had no blood work done the last six months. … We will get some blood work done.

I last saw Patient G in my office in mid-July 2015, more than 4 years after his first visit. Patient G remains fully compliant with his therapy, continues doing well, and continues enjoying his work, his life, and his family. He remains grateful to the therapy we offer. His blood sugars had been falling steadily in the range of 120 mg/dL in the mornings, ideal for him, rising only slightly throughout the day. He was on the lowest doses of insulin since starting treatment with me.

He described his 2-job routine as demanding, but he felt so well he had no problem meeting his responsibilities. His career, in fact, seemed to be going quite well, better than ever. He and his wife had purchased a new larger home, but even the stress of selling his old house and moving he handled without difficulty. I doubt in this particular case that Patient G will ever be free of all supplemental insulin, because he experienced such a catastrophic injury to his pancreas in 2007. However, I have learned not to underestimate the ability of any organ, even a very damaged one, to regenerate at least to some extent. In any event, Patient G continues experimenting with lowering his insulin dose, with ongoing success in improving his blood sugar regulation. As a final note to Patient G's complex history before his doctors finally diagnosed diabetes, repeated extensive blood testing did not show elevated blood sugars for 2.5 years.

CONCLUSION

Patient G provides an interesting example of how a precisely targeted, precisely prescribed diet designed according to a patient's autonomic state can lead to substantial improvement in serious illnesses other than cancer. In this case, in contradiction to current recommendations in both the conventional and more alternative medical worlds, Patient G's specific diet recommended a considerable daily intake of carbohydrates, though mostly complex, always as part of a whole food, and always from organic sources. In this way, along with the complementary supplement protocol, we were able—at least in our model of physiology—to reduce his sympathetic tone, increase parasympathetic firing, and increase β-cell activation and his own insulin production with resulting significant improvement not only in his blood sugars but also in his overall health.

REFERENCES

1. Gonzalez NJ, Isaacs LL. *The Trophoblast and the Origins of Cancer. One Solution to the Medical Enigma of our Time.* New York, NY: New Spring Press; 2009.

2. Ross CA. The trophoblast model of cancer. *Nutr Cancer.* 2015;67(1):61-67.

3. Gonzalez NJ, Isaacs LL. Evaluation of pancreatic proteolytic enzyme treatment of adenocarcinoma of the pancreas with nutrition and detoxification support. *Nutr Cancer.* 1999;33(2):117-124.

4. Chabot JA, Tsai WY, Fine RL, et al. Pancreatic proteolytic enzyme therapy compared with gemcitabine-based chemotherapy for the treatment of pancreatic cancer. *J Clin Oncol.* 2010;28(12):2058-2063.

5. Gonzalez NJ. *What Went Wrong: The Truth Behind the Clinical Trial of the Enzyme Treatment of Cancer.* New York, NY: New Spring Press; 2012.

6. Ross CA. Methodological flaws in the Chabot trial of pancreatic enzymes for pancreatic cancer. *Int J Cancer Prev Res.* 2015;1:1-4.

7. Pottenger FM. *Symptoms of Visceral Disease: A Study of The Vegetative Nervous System in Its Relationship to Clinical Medicine.* New York, NY: CV Mosby; 1922.

8. Gellhorn E. *Autonomic Imbalance and the Hypothalamus: Implications for Physiology, Medicine, Psychology, and Neuropsychiatry.* Minneapolis, MN: University of Minnesota Press; 1957.

9. Gonzalez NJ. *One Man Alone: An Investigation of Nutrition, Cancer, and William Donald Kelley.* New York, NY: New Spring Press; 2010.

10. Howell E. *Enzyme Nutrition.* New York, NY: Avery Publishing Group; 1995.

11. Oster K. *Homogenized Milk and Atherosclerosis.* Lawrence, KS: Sunflower Publishing; 1970.

12. Marshall JK, Thompson CE. Colon irrigation in the treatment of mental disease. *N Engl J Med.* September 1932;207:454-457.

The History of the Enzyme Treatment of Cancer

Nicholas Gonzalez, MD

Although there exists some debate over who discovered pancreatic enzymes, it appears the French physician Lucien Corvisart first described trypsin in 1856. However, the German researcher Julius Kühne deserves credit for actually naming this protease in 1876 and for introducing the concept of digestive enzymes as catalysts secreted by the pancreas that allow for efficient breakdown of food in the gastrointestinal (GI) tract.

By 1900, the 3 main classes of pancreatic enzymes had been identified: (1) the proteases that cleave proteins into constituent amino acids and peptides; (2) the amylases that reduce complex carbohydrates into simple disaccharides and trisaccharides; and (3) the lipases, which convert triglycerides into monoglycerides, diglycerides, and free fatty acids. Physiologists at the time, aware these enzymes worked best in a slightly alkaline environment, discovered that the pancreas released these various ferments, as they were called, into the duodenum during meals along with bicarbonate to neutralize the acidic chyme arriving from the stomach.

By the late 1800s, there was a flurry of activity among European researchers searching for therapeutic applications for the newly discovered enzymes, above and beyond any purely digestive use. Scientists discovered that trypsin could be useful in the treatment of diphtheria when applied directly to the tough fibrous membrane formed in the throat that could, if unchecked, lead to suffocation. In an animal model of the disease, a preparation of trypsin applied in the larynx appeared to digest away this tissue and when tested in humans, the enzyme worked quite well. An early reference to the successful treatment in humans dates from the October 23, 1886 issue of the *Journal of the American Medical Association*.[1]

In response to these early successes, by 1900, 2 pharmaceutical firms, Merck and the New York–based Fairchild, affiliated with Burroughs Wellcome, marketed powdered trypsin preparations derived from animal sources for treatment of the disease as well as injectable preparations for a hoped-for systemic effect. In addition, preparations meant for oral ingestion as a digestive aid became available, the most widely prescribed known as Holadin.

In 1902, the English scientist John Beard, DSc (1858-1924), Professor at the University of Edinburgh in Scotland, first proposed an anticancer activity for trypsin. His thesis, which would generate considerable controversy at the time, represented the culmination of some 20 years of meticulous research that began with the development of the nervous system in invertebrates.

Beard was not a physician but a zoologist trained as an embryologist: His graduate studies at the University of Freiburg in Germany, from which he received his doctoral degree in 1884, dealt with the embryogenesis of the sense organs in an obscure worm.[2] As his career evolved, he focused his attention on the developing nervous system of fish, then eventually mammals, and many of his pioneering findings from this period in his life, now proven correct, are standard fare in contemporary embryology texts.

It was Beard's study of the embryonic nervous system that, through a most convoluted route, led him to consider the formation and growth of the placenta, which anchors the mammalian fetus to the uterus and serves as the point of connection between the maternal blood vessels, providing oxygen and essential nutrients, and the blood of the embryo carrying the wastes of metabolism.

Beard was the first scientist to report that in many respects the placenta in its early stages—known as the trophoblast (from the Greek "to feed or nurture")—looks and behaves much like a cancer. Though we might think of the late 19th and early 20th centuries as a primitive time in medical research, by 1900 institutions devoted to cancer research, such as Sloan-Kettering in New York, were already up and running, with large staffs of scientists working to unravel the biology of cancer. By Beard's day, investigators had adeptly described the histology, behavior, and even the chromosome aberrations seen in the many varieties of malignant disease.

Cancer cells, it was well known at the time and as we agree today, possess certain well-defined characteristics. In appearance under a microscope, they display a primitive undifferentiated phenotype; in terms of behavior, they proliferate without restraint, can invade through tissue boundaries such as epithelial linings, and can migrate through organs while producing an extensive blood supply needed to support the characteristic exponential growth of malignancy.

Beard pointed out that the trophoblast begins as a very cancer-like tissue. It forms as an undifferentiated offshoot from the earliest stage of the embryo in the blastocyst phase, and its cells initially proliferate exponentially. The cells easily invade and migrate through the uterine epithelial lining and underlying stroma (an ability not seen in any other tissue except cancer) while, like a tumor, generating a rich blood vessel connection to the uterine maternal arteries and veins needed to maintain embryonic life. In terms of the last point, though the word *angiogenesis* is a modern term, Beard and his colleagues understood the concept quite well: the need for both tumors and the trophoblast to stimulate new vessel formation to allow for survival.

Beard was not only the first to note the similarities between the trophoblast and cancer, he went a huge step further in his thinking, claiming that cancer, whatever the histologic type, is fundamentally trophoblastic in its actual cellular origins. In laboratory experiments with animals, Beard found that during embryogenesis, many of the cells of the early trophoblast do not end up within the placenta itself but migrate throughout the various developing tissues and organs of the fetus to form undifferentiated nests that remain in place for the duration of the organism's life. Should these misplaced trophoblast cells be stimulated into reproductive activity through inflammation or infection, in the wrong place and at the wrong time, they become the invasive, exponentially growing tissue we identify as cancer.

Not surprisingly, Beard's scientific colleagues of 110 years ago could make no sense out of what he was saying, because no one else could identify these misplaced, "vagrant trophoblasts," as Beard called them, nor understand how they could form a cancer. Scientists believed then, as they were to believe for most of the 20th century, that cancer develops from mature differentiated cells in a tissue or organ that through some elaborate metamorphosis revert to a primitive morphology. In the process, these cells develop the hallmarks of cancer not seen in normal healthy tissues: an undifferentiated phenotype, unlimited proliferative potential, the ability to invade through tissue boundaries such as the basement membranes of epithelial linings, the ability to migrate through dense underlying stroma, the ability to metastasize, and the necessary ability to rapidly produce an ever-growing blood supply.

From a contemporary perspective, Beard, though discounted in his lifetime, may have been correct on all points. Scientists such as Murray and Lessey[3] at the University of North Carolina, and Ferretti[4] in Europe, have rediscovered the placental trophoblast as the ideal model for the study of cancer morphology, behavior, and molecular biology. As it turns out, cancer uses the same molecular mechanisms, the same transcription factors to turn genes on and off, and the same matrix metalloproteinases to invade through tissue boundaries and stroma as does the trophoblast. Further, those nests of primitive cells located in our various tissues Beard claimed to have identified were most likely what we today call stem cells. The concept of stem cells wouldn't enter our modern scientific consciousness until some 40 plus years after Beard's death, when in the 1960s McCulloch and Till,[5] evidently unaware of Beard's earlier work, would claim the discovery of these nests of undifferentiated cells that we now know are necessary for life. They provide an essential reservoir to replace cells lost due to normal turnover along the intestinal tract—which sloughs off every 5 days—or those lost due to injury, disease, or apoptosis.

As further confirmation of Beard's hypothesis, beginning in 2002 with Dr Wicha's work at the University of Michigan,[6-9] scientists at multiple institutions have been demonstrating that cancer does not develop as so long thought from mature, differentiated healthy cells that suddenly go molecularly berserk, transforming into the undifferentiated, invasive tissue of cancer. Instead, these investigators are showing rather convincingly that cancer develops from stem cells that lose their normal regulatory restraint.

Be that as it may, Beard well knew that in its normal timeline of growth, the trophoblast differed in 1 key regard from a cancerous tumor. At a specific point after conception—Beard claimed day 56 in humans—the trophoblast normally abruptly changes from a poorly differentiated, rapidly proliferating, invading, angiogenic tissue into the mature, highly differentiated, nonproliferating, noninvasive placenta. In its final incarnation, the placenta, a circular plate-like organ imbedded within the uterus some 8 to 10 inches in diameter and 1 to 2 inches thick, consists of a variety of well-differentiated cell types with minimal reproductive and no invasive potential. Thin-walled septa divide the placenta into sections like slices of a pie, with the mother's blood percolating on one side and the embryo's on the other.

In Beard's mind, the transformation of the early cancer-like trophoblast into the mature placenta was quite a remarkable biological feat, a process that became an obsession for him. Because he believed that cancer was not only *like* the trophoblast in its microscopic appearance and behavior, but was trophoblastic in its origins, he assumed if he could determine the factor or factors responsible for the change in trophoblastic character as the placenta formed, he would have the solution to cancer.

After years of research, Beard came to the conclusion that the key was in the embryonic pancreas. As witnessed in every mammalian species he studied, the very day the trophoblastic placenta converted from a poorly differentiated, invading tissue into the mature placenta, the embryonic pancreas began synthesizing and secreting its coterie of digestive enzymes. Contemporary molecular biologists have confirmed that the fetal pancreas does become active approximately when the trophoblast begins transforming into the mature placenta.[10,11]

Because it seemed pancreatic enzymes regulated trophoblast development, Beard logically assumed these same "ferments," in addition to their well-characterized digestive function, must be our main defense against cancer, keeping the "vagrant trophoblasts" in control, and would in turn also be useful as a cancer *treatment*.

After announcing his "trophoblastic theory of cancer" in a *Lancet* article in 1902,[12] Beard would first test his thesis in an animal tumor model available at the time, the Jensen's mouse tumor, what appears to have been a sarcoma-like malignancy. With 6 untreated tumor-laden mice as controls, after Dr Beard injected an extract of trypsin into 2 mice growing such cancers, the tumors completely regressed.[13] Subsequently, during the mid and later part of the first decade of the 20th century, a number of physicians interested in Beard's hypothesis began, under his direction, to use injectable pancreatic enzymes to treat their human cancer patients. The first report I have been able to locate, appearing in the *Medical Record* in November 1906 and written by New York physician Clarence Rice, was entitled "Treatment of Cancer of the Larynx by Subcutaenous Injection of Pancreatic Extract (Trypsin)" with the subtitle "A Case of Growth, Supposed to Be Carcinoma, Cured."[14] The history and results in this case with enzyme treatment were, in the author's estimation, "a remarkable cure." As an aside, Dr Rice recommended the Fairchild injectable preparation along with the oral supplement "Holadin."[14]

A month later, in December 1906, another New York physician, Margaret Cleaves, described 2 patients in the *Medical Record,* the first a woman with a recurrent large tumor of the tongue that stabilized on the enzyme treatment.[15] At the time of the publication, the patient had not been on the therapy very long but seemed to be improving substantially. The second case, a man with a large inoperable rectal carcinoma, experienced tumor necrosis, tumor liquefaction, and finally its sloughing off with the trypsin injections. Other case reports of successfully treated patients appeared in the major medical journals of the day, including the *Journal of the American Medical Association*[16] and the *British Medical Journal,*[17] describing apparent cures of patients diagnosed with head and neck, inoperable uterine, colorectal, and metastatic breast cancers.

During his lifetime, Dr Beard recommended only injectable preparations of pancreatic enzymes as a cancer treatment, assuming that for his specific purposes, orally ingested preparations would be of little value. It was generally believed then—as is still believed today—that trypsin, like any other protein ingested by mouth, would be degraded by the hydrochloric acid present in the stomach. Any active trypsin molecules that might survive this initial assault would then be subjected to autodigestion within the alkaline duodenum. Even if some trypsin did remain beyond this point, scientists already knew the protease to be a fairly large molecule that, they believed, could not possibly pass through the intestinal mucosa for systemic effect. In his classic textbook of the day, *Collected Contributions on Digestion and Diet,* the eminent physiologist Sir William Roberts, MD, made the case that orally ingested pancreatic enzymes would not survive very long in the digestive tract.[18]

By 1907, the initial successes reported in the literature generated considerable interest in Beard's enzyme treatment of cancer. In response to this enthusiasm, a growing number of firms began selling their own "trypsin" specifically as a cancer treatment in addition to those available from Merck and Fairchild. With trypsin formulations widely available, physicians both in the United States and in Europe began applying the therapy, usually without consulting Beard, and with variable results. As both positive and negative reports began to filter into the literature, Beard began to suspect that many of the available preparations had little potency and, hence, little efficacy.[19]

From our readings in the literature, it seems that in Beard's era, the manufacturers used a very simple process to extract the enzymes, first mincing the glands in cold water, pressing the mixture, then removing the active component with an alcohol solvent. The alcohol would then be allowed to evaporate off, leaving the desired enzyme fraction.[20] However, pancreatic enzymes are quite unstable over time in an aqueous environment, prone to autodigestion. We suspect the procedure used in Beard's day was neither exacting nor refined, the final preparation, most likely, containing little in the way of potential enzyme activity. To make matters worse, those products intended for injectable use were provided in solution in vial form, an ideal environment for the autodigestion process to begin. Fairchild did market a dry powdered "trypsin" meant to be mixed with water immediately before injection, but even this proved so unstable that by 1907, as Beard reported, the company discontinued its sale.[12]

In the November 16, 1907 issue of the *Lancet*, P. Tetens Hald, MD, "Formerly Assistant in the Pharmacological Institute of the University of Copenhagen" and a Beard proponent, published the results of his evaluation of 6 popular enzyme products available at the time, including those marketed by Merck and Fairchild.[21] In his research, he employed the same method used today to assess proteolytic activity, the casein digestion test. This simple assay measures the amount of the milk protein casein curdled over time by a known quantity of pancreas product.

Dr Hald contacted the manufacturers of the various products he analyzed in his laboratory, none of whom provided him with any information about the stability of the formulations they sold commercially. To his surprise, his assays revealed the potencies varied enormously, up to a factor of 400, and that the activity levels rarely correlated with the company's claims, as stated on the bottle or in its literature.[21]

In his 1911 book *The Enzyme Treatment of Cancer*, Dr Beard himself bemoaned the dearth of standardized and potent enzyme preparations, a situation that led to inevitable treatment failures when physicians used products of poor quality. He actually quoted a Merck publication from the time, in which the writer discussed the confusion in the field:

> The actual position of affairs in the past few years can best be described by quoting the impartial opinion of a competent author. On p. 340 of *E. Merck's Annual Report of Recent Advances in Pharmaceutical Chemistry and Therapeutics* (Darmstadt, vol. xxii., August, 1909) one may read regarding trypsin: "The mode of action and the value of pancreas preparations in cancer has not yet received a wholly reliable explanation. Great difficulties are encountered because the preparations used by the various investigators differ greatly in respect to their chemical properties, their purity, and in the amount of active substances they contain, and often these factors are not fully known to the student of the literature, or to the physician who has used them and describes their action. Further difficulties arise when pancreatin [whole pancreas product] and trypsin are described as substances of equal value, and how shall we gauge the action of pancreatin

and trypsin ampullae whose mode of preparation and whose composition is not mentioned in the original paper, neither is there any mention made of their sterility or the method by which they have been sterilized? ... So long as the solutions of pancreatin and trypsin are treated as secret remedies no one will be able to form a clear picture of the value of trypsin treatment from the many publications which have appeared."[12]

In reference to the above, as an aside we find it interesting that by 1909, Beard's hypothesis had generated interest sufficient enough to warrant thoughtful discussion in the annual report of a major international pharmaceutical company. This exposition also supports Beard's contention that the mixed results for enzyme treatment being reported in the literature most likely reflected no flaw in the theory, only variations in the quality of product.

Despite the initial enthusiasm for Beard's trophoblastic hypothesis and the clinical enzyme treatment, ultimately the medical community at large seemed to have mobilized an angry backlash against Beard and his followers. He was attacked in medical journals and newspapers, and he was belittled at scientific conventions. Nonetheless, Dr Beard stuck to his course and fought back in articles and letters to the editor, and in *The Enzyme Treatment of Cancer*, a text that outlined his years of research and the promising laboratory and clinical results.[12] Regardless, interest in Beard's thesis gradually petered out, and when he died in 1924, he died frustrated, angry, and ignored, his therapy already considered no more than an historical oddity.

Though the rejection of something new in the scientific research community hardly seems surprising—it is of course the historical norm—I find the ultimate indifference toward, and contempt for, Dr Beard evident in his contemporary academic colleagues most unfortunate. Beard was, after all, an impeccably trained scientist, a professor at an eminent European university whose embryological findings are still accepted in the texts of our day. He carefully documented his laboratory and clinical results that he published in the conventional medical literature. But it seems to have made no difference at all.

A number of factors contributed to the decline of interest after 1911 in Dr Beard's trophoblastic hypothesis and his enzyme approach to cancer. Certainly, the enthusiasm for the X-ray, discovered in 1895 by Röntgen, helped push Beard's treatment into the background.[22] After all, at the same time Beard was arguing his case, 2-time Nobel Laureate Marie Curie, widely admired and respected at all levels of society, had vigorously championed the mysterious invisible rays as a nontoxic cure for all cancer, a breakthrough the press promoted with great enthusiasm. Beard, on the other hand, had no such media savvy science star to praise his ideas about the use of enzymes against malignant disease. And it would not be until after Beard's death in 1924 that researchers began to appreciate the severe limitations of radiation treatment, which in reality worked well against only a few cancers. Even for those tumors that did respond initially, usually the disease recurred with a vengeance and the therapy once thought to be harmless, actually as all physicians know today, could be quite toxic. An entire generation of radiation researchers died as a result of cavalier exposure to the rays, including Marie Curie herself who eventually succumbed to radiation-induced aplastic anemia.[24] By then, Beard was long forgotten.

Above and beyond the realities of scientific politics, we suspect that poor quality enzyme products did much to undermine Beard's treatment. In a sense, Beard was a victim of his own fame. The initial successes reported in the literature prompted many doctors to begin using any number of enzyme formulations without first consulting Beard about dosing and quality, with inevitable poor or mixed results. The disappointments fueled the criticism in the journals, to the point that after 1911, few doctors of Beard's generation even considered the treatment for their patients.[25]

Though interest in Beard's cancer treatment dwindled, certainly after his death, injectable formulations of pancreatic enzymes remained available in the United States and Europe for treatment of diphtheria, along with oral preparations intended for treatment of digestive problems and pancreatic insufficiency.

By the 1940s, the commercial demand for pancreatic enzymes such as trypsin had expanded greatly beyond their limited pharmaceutical applications. For example, leather tanners used proteolytic enzymes to speed up curing, and candy manufacturers learned that trypsin, when added during the processing of chocolate, helped create a smoother product.

But the commercial suppliers still relied on the old mincing and alcohol method of extracting proteolytic enzymes from the animal gland, a very inefficient technique that gave a 10% to 15% yield.[20] A potential bonanza awaited anyone who might develop a more efficient enzyme purification process.

The biochemist Ezra Levin of Champaign, Illinois, active during the 1940s and 1950s and at the time one of the leading experts in the manufacture of pancreatic enzymes, believed he had done just that. His lengthy 1950 US patent entitled "Production of Dried, Defatted Enzymatic Material" detailed his crowning achievement, an elaborate multistep process for extracting active enzymes from the gland that he insisted was more efficient and more cost-effective than the previous methodology.[20] During his process, all fat, which he saw as waste, would be removed and importantly, most if not all the precursors such as trypsinogen would be activated, yielding a product of high potency with purported minimal processing losses—a product that Levin and his customers thought ideal for pharmaceutical as well as industrial use.

Levin had made 2 assumptions as he perfected his method. First, he believed that the fat in the gland—and the pancreas is a fatty gland—had no useful purpose beyond its role as a storage depot for excess calories and needed to be removed. To him, fat seemed little more than inert filler. Second, he always assumed the more activated the product, the better.[20]

Levin actually created a company, Viobin, for years a subsidiary of A. H. Robbins, to manufacture and market his enzyme products. The Levin method proved so successful that by the 1960s, Viobin provided most of the enzymes used in the United States, both for pharmaceutical and other industrial purposes. Even other manufacturers that ventured into the enzyme business themselves relied on variations of the Levin patent.

THE SALVATION OF AN IDEA

Though relegated to obscurity, during the 20th century, Beard's enzyme thesis did not disappear completely. Periodically, other physicians and scientists rediscovered his work, saw the potential benefit in his hypothesis, and kept the idea alive, however tenuously. During the 1920s and 1930s, a St Louis physician, Dr F. L. Morse, reported that he had successfully treated a number of advanced cancer patients with injectable pancreatic enzymes. When he presented his well-documented findings to the St Louis Medical Society in 1934—a proceeding published in the *Weekly Bulletin of the St. Louis Medical Society*—his colleagues attacked him viciously and relentlessly.[26] One physician at the session, a Dr M. G. Seelig, remarked, "While I heartily agree with Dr Allen when he strikes the note of encouragement, I recoil at the idea of witlessly spreading the hope of a cancer cure which is implicit in the remarks of Dr Morse this evening ..."

Subsequently, Frank Shively, MD, a Dayton, Ohio surgeon active during the 1960s,[27] rediscovered Beard's earlier papers and used injectable formulations of pancreatic enzymes in his treatment protocols. In a self-published 1969 monograph, *Multiple Proteolytic Enzyme Therapy of Cancer*, Dr Shively reported on 192 cases of patients diagnosed with advanced cancer treated with injectable enzymes, with 12 apparent "cures." However, in 1966, the Food and Drug Administration, perhaps in response to Shively's growing reputation, forbade the sale of injectable pancreatic enzymes, and the surgeon seemed to have returned to more mundane medical pursuits.

Contemporaneously with Dr Shively, in the 1960s, William Donald Kelley, DDS, first appeared on the scene, with his complex cancer treatment involving a whole foods diet, large amounts of various nutritional supplements, detoxification routines such as coffee enemas, and prodigious doses of pancreatic enzymes ingested orally—but never injected.

Kelley claimed he discovered the anticancer properties of oral pancreatic enzymes without any previous knowledge of Dr Beard. Kelley had been a successful orthodontist with a serious interest in nutrition, practicing in Grapevine, Texas, when in the early 1960s, while he was only in his mid-30s, he became devastatingly ill. His doctors eventually diagnosed advanced pancreatic cancer, though he never underwent tissue sampling—not uncommon in the days before computerized tomography (CT) scans and core biopsies. In desperation, with 4 children dependent on him, Kelley through trial and error devised his own nutritional program to slow the disease, including an organic, largely vegetarian raw foods diet, a variety of supplements, and the coffee enemas. He also added high doses of oral pancreatic enzymes to his regimen, not because of any familiarity with Beard's hypothesis, but to help relieve his severe digestive distress—as occurs commonly in patients with pancreatic malignancy.

Kelley's digestion was so poor, he began ingesting huge amounts of pancreatin around the clock hoping to keep his worsening symptoms—including excruciating pain whenever he ate—at bay. He discovered that with large doses, his tolerance for food improved and, to his surprise, his large tumors, readily palpable through the abdominal wall, seemed to regress. Perplexed by his observations, he scoured the medical literature looking for evidence that someone else might have witnessed an anticancer effect for pancreatic enzymes. His search eventually led him to Dr Beard's book and papers from 50 years earlier, but by that point, as he claimed, Kelley had already worked out the rudiments of his treatment.

From that very personal experience began Kelley's foray out of conventional orthodontics into the controversial world of nutritional cancer therapeutics. By the late 1960s, having long abandoned dentistry, he refocused his attention on treating, with his nutritional regimen, the very ill drawn from all over the country, most diagnosed with advanced malignancy. With the publication of his 1969 book *One Answer to Cancer*,[28] Kelley for better or worse secured his position as a preeminent alternative cancer therapist and inevitably as a target for the mainstream medical world which then, as now, had little use for proposed nutritional approaches to the disease.

Kelley intently studied the writings of Beard, who strongly insisted the treatment needed to be applied via injection. Nonetheless, for the duration of his career, Kelley only recommended oral formulations. Though injectable preparations were still available in the United States during the early years of Kelley's nutritional practice, as a dentist, Kelley lacked the legal right to prescribe injectable enzymes. Even if such products had remained on the market and even if he had the authority to use them, his own experience treating himself, and his subsequent experience with hundreds of patients taught him that oral preparations worked very well.

I met Dr Kelley by chance during the summer following my second year of medical school in 1981. At that time, he seemed completely modest and unassuming, seeking only to have his work properly evaluated so that if the approach had merit, it might become more widely accessible to patients in need. I was fortunate to have as a mentor at Cornell Medical College the late Robert A. Good, MD, PhD, then president of the Sloan-Kettering Research Institute, who encouraged a review of Kelley's cases.

Under Dr Good's direction, I began a student project evaluating Dr Kelley's patients, methods, successes, and failures. During a rather extraordinary summer spent reading through Kelley's records in his main Dallas office, I quickly found evidence of what appeared to be patient after patient with appropriately diagnosed, biopsy proven advanced and even terminal cancer, who were alive 5, even 10 years since first beginning the enzyme therapy. What began as a mere student investigation eventually evolved into a full-fledged research project, completed while I was a fellow in Dr Good's group, which, after he left Sloan, moved first to the University of Oklahoma, then to All Children's Hospital in Florida.

As part of my project, I eventually interviewed and evaluated more than 1000 of Kelley's patients, concentrating on a group of some 455 patients diagnosed with cancer who had done well under his care. From this population, I wrote up in detail 50 cases, representing 26 different types of cancer. Even today, nearly 30 years later, I am still impressed by Kelley's achievement. For example, one of these patients, a woman who ran a gas station with her husband in Wisconsin, was diagnosed in August 1982 with metastatic adenocarcinoma of the pancreas, the worst form, with biopsy-proven metastases into the liver. The Mayo Clinic confirmed the diagnosis, offered no treatment, and told her she might live 12 months. With no conventional options recommended, she began looking into alternative approaches, learned of Kelley, and began his treatment.

I first interviewed her in 1986, 4 years after her diagnosis, as part of my Kelley investigation. At the time, still following her nutritional regimen, she reported feeling quite well. In the many years since, we have kept in touch regularly and today in 2014, she is alive, well, and as feisty as ever, now 32 years from her original diagnosis. She has never returned to her conventional physicians for follow-up radiographic studies, but to put her case in perspective, I have searched the literature repeatedly and know of no other similar patient with biopsy-proven liver metastases from pancreatic adenocarcinoma documented at a major institution, alive and well 32 years later.

Another patient was initially diagnosed with adenocarcinoma of the uterus in 1969. Because of the large size of the tumor, her doctors advised a course of intensive radiation therapy before hysterectomy. Because her doctors thought the disease was localized, postoperatively no adjuvant therapy was suggested.

However, by 1974, her general health had deteriorated significantly; she experienced unrelenting fatigue, severe depression, weight loss, and vague abdominal pains. Initially her physicians attributed her symptoms to "nerves," but when she developed a grapefruit-sized tumor in her pelvis, she was referred back to her surgeon. At that time, an X-ray revealed multiple tumors in both lungs consistent with metastatic disease. Her surgeon recommended palliative resection of the pelvic tumor nonetheless to prevent an impending intestinal obstruction, though he admitted to the patient she had an incurable disease. Subsequently, she underwent the suggested surgery then consulted with an oncologist who prescribed a synthetic progesterone, which he explained might prolong her life. But the patient experienced such serious side effects, she discontinued the drug after some 6 weeks and with no further options began investigating alternative treatments for cancer. After learning of Dr Kelley, she consulted with him and followed her prescribed nutritional program religiously.

Under Kelley's care, her health gradually improved. She avoided all conventional doctors for a time, but 9 years after starting her regimen, in 1984, she returned to her former primary care physician for evaluation of an irregular heart rhythm, a long-standing problem. The physician, as the records indicate, was astonished she was still alive. A chest X-ray confirmed total resolution of her previously described multiple pulmonary nodules. Subsequently, she kept in touch with me periodically until her death in 2009 at age 95, 34 years after her diagnosis of metastatic disease, some 40 years from her original diagnosis. To put her case in perspective, I have searched the literature and know of no similar patient with recurrent endometrial cancer who experienced total regression of disease and survival of 34 years after the appearance of extensive metastases.

During my investigation of Kelley's therapy and patients, as a side project I also tried to evaluate the relative efficacy of the different pancreatic formulations he had recommended during his time in practice. By the time I met Kelley in 1981, he had become convinced that the more active the oral product, the better the effect against cancer, insisting as well he wanted no precursors in his formulation. I even traveled with Kelley to Wisconsin in the summer of 1981 to meet with the manufacturer he used at the time to discuss with them his new plans for the strongest supplement possible, containing only fully activated, and defatted, pancreatin.

From Kelley's records and our conversations about the issue, I had a fairly good idea of which strength of enzyme he used during which period, and from my review of his patient charts on a year-by-year basis, it seemed to me that his greatest success as a practitioner occurred during the period from 1970 to 1982, when he relied primarily on a modestly activated formulation containing a high percentage of inactive precursors. After he opted for increasingly more activated product, it seemed to me his success declined with the "stronger" preparation.

In any event, I finished my "Kelley Project" in 1986 and wrote up the results in monograph form hoping the unusual case reports would stimulate research interest in the therapy from academia. But despite Dr Good's support and 5 years of serious research efforts, I was unable to get the book published. Sadly, Kelley turned increasingly paranoid, at one point accusing me of being sent by the Central Intelligence Agency to steal his therapy for the government. He had shut down his practice and, after 1987, I had no further direct contact with Kelley. My monograph about Kelley's work was finally published in 2010 as *One Man Alone*, with a lengthy new introduction.[29]

When my colleague Dr Linda Isaacs and I arrived in New York in the fall of 1987 determined to salvage Kelley's treatment, we knew if we were to succeed in practice, we needed a reliable source of enzymes. As I thought about the situation, I realized we must determine the optimal composition for the enzyme product in terms of relative fat and protein content, as well as the ideal level of proteolytic activity—and hopefully find a source that met our specifications.

I had already begun to move away from the Levin methodology as the best for manufacturing pancreatic enzymes. I knew that he had designed his extraction method to remove as much fat as possible, which he perceived as useless filler. I thought in this regard, Levin, as well as Kelley who accepted without question Levin's dictates, had been wrong, and that fat might allow for a more stable product and provide physiological benefit. By 1987, researchers had already begun to suspect that fat was not just a simple warehouse for storing excess energy, but a metabolically active tissue secreting a variety of enzymes and hormones that regulate the processing of sugars and fatty acids. Perhaps, I thought, the lipid component of the pancreas might itself provide some additional effect, a complement to the proteolytic activity. So as a first order of business, I decided to search for an enzyme preparation containing significant fat.

Ezra Levin also assumed that the more active the product the better, the mantra Kelley again professed to me with total conviction. But I knew from my exhaustive evaluation of Kelley's files that as he opted for a more potent enzyme formulation, his response rate fell. In frustration, he assumed he only needed to prescribe an even stronger enzyme, or change encapsulators, etc, instead of retracing his steps and going backward to the less active 4× enzymes he had earlier used with great success.

I became convinced that as brilliant as Kelley had been in his prime, he had erred in his later years by assuming that "purer and more active" is always unquestionably better. I suspected that the fat-depleted, highly activated supplements may have been prone to deteriorate once encapsulated, susceptible to rapid autodigestion on the shelf. I also became convinced that the fat in the gland might not only help stabilize the mix, but provide synergistic factors to assist the proteolytic enzymes in their fight against malignant cells. Finally, I came to believe that an enzyme with less activity, with more of the total potential as precursor, might not only be more stable in the bottle, but more effective against cancer.

As a first order of business, I obtained samples of pancreatin from a number of suppliers who manufactured their own products. I also visited several health food stores and nutritional pharmacies in Manhattan, such as Willner Chemists, purchasing a variety of pancreatic enzyme supplements. In the kitchen of my mother's home in Queens where we were staying at the time, I set up my own enzyme assay, using Knox gelatin as my protein substrate instead of casein, and the Viobin preparation Viokase as my standard by which to measure the activity of other products. I dissolved each capsule or tablet in a slightly alkaline solution to help promote the enzymatic reactions and then observed the amount of gelatin digested over time. The assay, which I repeated many times for a number of weeks, worked quite well. Unfortunately, nearly all of the enzymes I tested seemed highly activated and highly processed, with all the fat removed.

Finally, I learned of the pancreas enzyme product derived from New Zealand pigs available from Allergy Research Group, a nutritional supplement company of some renown based in northern California. As a start, I was happy about the source, because I had learned that New Zealand had perhaps the cleanest environment of any country on Earth, as well as the strictest laws for raising animals for commercial use. Diseases such as hoof and mouth disease and trichinosis, I was told, had never been reported there.

I also wanted enzymes derived from the pig pancreas, thought to be most similar to the human organ. For decades, before the advent of genetically engineered preparations, physicians treated their diabetic patients with pig insulin, which proved to be quite similar in terms of amino acid structure to the human variety. In a similar manner, pig enzymes, I had learned from conversations with Viobin scientists, most closely resembled ours, of all commercially available sources.

Most important, the Allergy Research Group (ARG) specifications described their pancreas supplement as a freeze-dried product, minimally processed, *with the fat intact*, yet it still tested active at moderate levels by my own assay—exactly what we wanted. Though the material had not been intentionally activated as per Levin, I suspected during the handling of the glands, some of the precursors spontaneously converted, fortuitously to the precise level we thought ideal. Then, with freeze-drying complete, all activation would come to a halt, leaving a stable product with most of the proteolytic enzymes in the precursor form.

I contacted the founder of ARG, Dr Stephen Levine, and introduced myself, explaining my plan to open up a practice and my need for good quality enzymes. Though I was virtually unknown at the time, he agreed to provide me with as much of the product as we required. With a supply of enzymes guaranteed, in late 1987 we opened our practice with great optimism in an office in Manhattan. To our relief, this enzyme worked quite well, confirming my belief that a minimally processed lightly activated preparation, with the fat intact, was ideal for our purposes.

One of my first successes dated from December 1987, shortly after I had opened my practice in New York. A woman came to me with a diagnosis of aggressive inflammatory breast cancer that had metastasized to her bones while she was receiving chemotherapy. She had been first diagnosed in 1985 with a tumor so large she could not initially proceed with surgery. After 5 weeks of radiation to the breast to shrink the mass, she underwent mastectomy. Even after radiation, the tumor was still huge at 8 cm in widest diameter, and 17 of 17 axillary lymph nodes were involved with cancer, though there was no evidence of distant spread by radiographic studies. She then began chemotherapy with cyclophosphamide, methotrexate, and fluorouracil, which her doctors told her she would need to continue for the rest of her life, explaining that at some point the disease inevitably would recur. Unfortunately, after 2 years of treatment, in late 1987 a bone scan revealed multiple areas of activity consistent with widespread metastatic disease. At that point she consulted me, began the program with great dedication, and clinically improved. She refused any follow-up testing until some 14 years after she had begun treatment with me, when in 2001 a bone scan revealed total resolution of her disease. Today, more than 26 years from her diagnosis of metastatic inflammatory breast cancer, she remains alive, well, and cancer-free, still ingesting a fair amount of pancreatic enzymes.

We treated all our early successes, right up until 1995, with pancreatic enzymes available from ARG. Between 1995 and 1998, we entered into a research and development arrangement with Procter & Gamble, who generously provided extensive financial support as well as a team of scientists to help us determine definitively the best enzyme formulation for our purposes. The company spent considerable time, effort, and money evaluating our enzymes, even sending researchers to New Zealand to observe firsthand the entire processing of the pancreas glands from slaughterhouse to finished material. With such assistance, we eventually refined the methodology still further to help guarantee consistent manufacture of a stable, modestly active, minimally processed product with most of the enzymes—but not all—in the precursor form, and with a certain percentage of fat remaining. Working with our New Zealand supplier, we developed a method to help assure the desired potency with each batch, without the need for Levin's complicated system of fat extraction and vacuum distillation. Today, we still rely on that same enzyme preparation, which we find works even more effectively than our earlier supplement.

ORAL VERSUS INJECTABLE ENZYMES

In his 1897 text *Collected Contributions on Digestion and Diet*, Dr William Roberts reported his experiments "proving" that hydrochloric acid permanently inactivated pancreatic "ferments," as he called the enzymes, taken by mouth.[18] Beard knew of Roberts's writings, which he held in some esteem, even referencing him by name in his own book *The Enzyme Treatment of Cancer*.[12] Fully accepting Roberts's conclusions, Beard insisted that for any effect against cancer, the practitioner must administer the pancreas enzymes in an injectable form. Though Beard's proponents such as Dr Rice did prescribe oral preparations along with the injectable, these were intended strictly as supplemental, not as primary therapy.[14]

Today, 100 years later, most physiologists still cite the same mantra proposed by Roberts, claiming that pancreatic enzymes ingested orally cannot survive contact with hydrochloric acid in the stomach or autodigestion in the duodenum, nor could they ever be absorbed. Critics of our work proclaim that even if pancreatic enzymes do have an anticancer potential, our therapy as administered today can't possibly succeed because we prescribe oral formulations exclusively. When I lecture, often at the end someone will question the feasibility of systemic benefit with the oral supplements we recommend.

With all due respect to Dr Beard, physiologists, and critics, orally ingested pancreatic enzymes must survive digestive assault and be absorbed because in practice they work, as Kelley's successes and our own would attest. But if we put aside Kelley's experience or ours for a moment, a review of the scientific literature does not support the current dogma but long ago confirmed that pancreatic enzymes taken by mouth survive the gauntlet of the digestive tract and can be absorbed into the systemic circulation to a substantial degree.

The late physician Dr Edward Howell first investigated in some depth the absorption of orally ingested enzymes for possible therapeutic action during the first half of the 20th century. Howell was not an academic scientist but a practicing physician and independent researcher, best known as the grandfather of the current raw foods movement. Howell proposed decades ago that raw foodstuffs provide all the vitamins, minerals, trace elements, fibers, proteins, fats, and carbohydrates in an undamaged, optimal form allowing for greatest physiological benefit. Among these essentials, he also included enzymes present in our food, which he believed could be absorbed intact and active like a vitamin or mineral, to aid in normal metabolism and in repair of tissue damage.

In his clinical practice, Howell applied a variety of raw foods diets and enzyme supplements, claiming great success. Judging by his writings, he became rather expert not only in dietetics but in the field of enzymes, their therapeutic use, and in particular their absorption when taken by mouth. In his 1946 book, *The Status of Food Enzymes in Digestion and Metabolism*, later reprinted as *Food Enzymes for Health & Longevity*,[30] he reviewed the literature on enzyme therapeutics to that time. Surprisingly enough, he seems to have been totally ignorant of Dr Beard's thesis from 40 years earlier.

Despite that oversight, in a chapter entitled "Intestinal Absorbability of Enzymes," Dr Howell argued the case from the scientific literature that pancreatic enzymes specifically ingested as supplements survive digestion to be absorbed from the intestinal tract into both the bloodstream as well as the lymphatic system.[30]

His well-referenced document, though old, makes interesting reading from a historical perspective. When I first studied the book, I was surprised to learn that even by 1946, a considerable body of evidence indicated large proteins in general, and pancreatic enzymes in particular, taken by mouth did end up in the general circulation. In the following, Howell discussed the findings from a group of Japanese researchers who evaluated the levels of enzymes in urine over a 24-hour period after an oral challenge:

> What I believe is one of the most outstanding researches so far recorded on the fate of enzymes when taken orally was undertaken by Masumizu, Medical Clinic, Tohoku Imperial University, Japan. Masumizu's work is remarkable in several ways. The experiments were conducted, not upon isolated specimens of urine, but upon the complete 24 hour excretion, thereby insuring the presence of all enzymes excreted, instead of only a portion. The experimental animals, 10 rabbits, were given by os [mouth], 5 grams of pancreatin or 5 grams of fungus amylase for each rabbit per day. Since this dosage is comparatively enormous for small animals, the experiments prove beyond doubt that even large quantities of enzymes can be absorbed and find their way into the urine.[30]

In more recent times, the published literature again confirms that orally ingested enzymes can survive exposure to hydrochloric acid in the stomach, the alkaline environment of the duodenum, and be absorbed efficiently through the small intestinal mucosa.

We will address the first point, the denaturation of pancreatic enzymes by stomach acid. An article by Moskvichyov et al[31] of the All-Union Scientific Research Technological Institute of Antibiotics and Enzymes for Medical Applications, published in *Enzyme Microbiology and Technology* in 1988, discussed this very issue in some detail. The authors begin by reviewing the previously published data, which rather conclusively demonstrated the stability of trypsin exposed to high temperatures even in the presence of acid:

> In the first reports by J.H. Northrop, J. Mellanby and V.J. Woolley on heating trypsin in dilute acid solutions up to boiling point it was demonstrated that activity loss was minimal. The unusual property of trypsin, i.e. its high thermostability, was not clearly understood then. The most interesting and promising reports did not appear until the late 1960s, when the kinetics of the reverse denaturation of trypsin and chymotrypsin were described. It was then established that the unusual properties of these proteinases are due to the conformational transitions between different states of the protein molecule while the equilibrium between them may shift, depending upon external conditions.[31]

Moskvichyov et al[31] describe their own elaborate experiments proving stability of trypsin even when exposed to acid at high temperatures. The authors demonstrated that in a solution of heated acid, active trypsin exists in a dynamic equilibrium with its denatured configuration. With higher heat and greater acid concentration, the reaction favors the denatured form; with cooling and a more alkaline pH, the process yields more of the active trypsin. In this system, the inactive conformation, apparently protected from damage, can convert, as pH goes up and temperature drops, back into the functional enzyme. This work proves that trypsin denaturation by heat or acid is *not permanent but a reversible process*—thus contradicting the basic assumptions of many.

Therefore, orally ingested pancreatic enzyme preparations should easily survive the hydrochloric acid present in the stomach. In the next assumed obstacle, the alkaline liquid environment of the duodenum, the enzymes become most active—and most susceptible, the experts teach, to autodigestion. Few of these molecules, they claim, could possibly survive this drive to mass molecular suicide.

Once again, contrary to tradition, the evidence shows that pancreatic enzymes including trypsin, lipase, and amylase survive the duodenal environment largely intact and active. In a 1975 study, Legg and Spencer[32] reported their experiences with the 3 enzymes stored for 4 weeks in alkaline human duodenal juice at various temperatures. All 3 seemed fairly stable kept at -20°C, with 85% of the trypsin retained in its active state. At 5°C, 70% of the trypsin remained potent. At room temperature, losses were more substantial, though even after 4 days, 70% of trypsin remained viable, a rather substantial amount. Clearly, pancreatic enzymes appear stable in duodenal juices, even at room temperature, even for a considerable period of time.

Contemporary critics have long proclaimed the third obstacle, the improbable absorption of pancreatic enzymes through the intestinal mucosa, as the most daunting, in their minds precluding any systemic benefit from orally ingested preparations. In the standard teaching, with each meal the pancreas must pour out a substantial quantity of newly minted enzymes, which will gradually digest themselves away along with the food. This scenario requires that the gland must continually synthesize enormous amounts of all enzymes in constant preparation for the next meal, 24 hours a day, for the lifetime of the organism.[33]

Yet again, the actual scientific data contradict cherished traditions. Over the past 3 decades, the physiologists Charles Liebow, currently at the State University of New York at Buffalo, and who taught at Cornell Medical College during my days there, and Stephen Rothman, of the University of California, San Francisco, have investigated the absorption of activated pancreatic enzymes as well as their precursors.

In their long years of research, these 2 investigators focused on the recycling of pancreatic enzymes secreted into the intestinal tract during digestion. As their first premise, they thought it impossible that the pancreas could create the copious enzyme supply needed for each meal de novo as experts have long assumed. In a series of elegant experiments they demonstrated that contrary to accepted dogma, the enzyme load secreted by the pancreas during meals is not destroyed but instead largely reabsorbed and recycled, in what they refer to as an "enteropancreatic" process, akin to the enterohepatic recirculation of bile salts.

In an early article on the subject entitled "Enteropancreatic Circulation of Digestive Enzymes," published in *Science* in 1975, Liebow and Rothman[34] reported

Gonzalez—History of Enzyme Treatment for Cancer

on the absorption of enzymes both in laboratory models as well as in live animals. They conclude that the enzymes easily pass through the intestinal mucosa:

> Digestive enzyme in the blood can be derived from at least two sources—the acinar cell itself and from the intestinal lumen via the bloodstream. The intestinal epithelium is permeable to a variety of proteins; for digestive enzymes in particular, substantial elastase, chymotrypsin, and trypsin permeabilities have been reported. We examined chymotrypsinogen permeability by comparing the mucosal to serosal flux of [³H] chymotrypsinogen relative to that for [¹³¹I]albumin across gut sacs prepared from rabbit ileum … nevertheless, we found that the permeability of the ileal membrane to chymotrypsinogen expressed per unit of concentration gradient was some nine times greater than that found for albumin …
>
> The existence of an enteropancreatic circulation for at least some digestive enzymes seems clear.[34]

Not surprising, their initial findings met with strong resistance from fellow physiologists, who despite the formidable evidence stuck to the old belief that pancreatic enzymes cannot be absorbed through the intestinal lining. To their credit, Liebow and Rothman[33] continued their studies, eventually summarizing their experience as well as the controversy still lingering over their findings in a lengthy review article entitled "Conservation of Digestive Enzymes" appearing in the January 2002 issue of *Physiology Reviews*. Their article begins:

> In this review we summarize experiments whose implications were of great interest when they were first reported. They provided unexpected evidence that the conventional belief that every meal is digested by an entirely new complement of digestive enzymes is incorrect. The data suggested that instead of being completely degraded in the small bowel with the food they digest, a large fraction of the digestive enzymes secreted by the pancreas are absorbed and recycled in an enteropancreatic circulation.[33]

The authors then proceed to catalogue in some detail the results of their experiments over the years, before essentially demolishing their critics. After some 16 pages, they conclude:

> As we reexamined the evidence for a conservation of digestive enzymes, we found it no less compelling than we did 25 years ago. Likewise, we found the studies that question its existence as incomplete as they seemed to us all those years ago …
>
> The traditional single pass view of digestion in which a completely new complement of digestive enzymes is manufactured for each meal has the curious consequence of requiring the organism to be particularly wasteful in its expenditure of energy to manufacture these costly molecules to meet its needs for sustenance … when just the opposite would seem desirable.[33]

Liebow and Rothman thus show that pancreatic enzymes present in the small intestine don't self-destruct but survive to be largely and efficiently assimilated into the bloodstream for reuse. Though the 2 researchers have specifically studied the fate of enzymes secreted into the duodenum by the pancreas, the same rule presumably holds true for enzymes provided in supplement form.

To summarize, orally ingested pancreatic enzymes may easily survive the alleged ravages of hydrochloric acid in the stomach, the alkaline environment of the duodenum, and can then pass into the systemic circulation, with little loss along the way. The scientific documentation as reported in the literature therefore suggests that oral preparations can have a systemic effect as we have witnessed in our practice for some 27 years.

As a final point, I had observed, in my review of Kelley's patient charts, that a modestly activated product with most of the enzymes in precursor form worked best. In our own practice beginning in 1987, we found such a formulation seemed to work quite efficiently, though we were not sure on a molecular level why this might be the case, particularly because Kelley had strongly argued for a highly activated supplement. It was not until we became aware, in 2005, of the research of Novak and Trnka[35] that we finally discovered a rationale for our less activated product. In their excellent article "Proenzyme Therapy of Cancer," the authors, very much aware of Dr Beard's work, surmise that the injectable formulations he recommended for treatment unbeknownst to him most likely provided a high percentage of precursors.[35] The authors point out that Beard always insisted that for best results, the pancreatin must be prepared from fresh animal glands quickly processed, material that would provide most of the enzymes in their inactive conformation. Though Beard always identified trypsin as the primary anticancer enzyme, Novak and Trnka insist the proenzymes such as trypsinogen and not the active configurations provided benefit in Beard's investigations.

In their own animal and human studies, Novak and Trnka[35] discovered that a pancreatin consisting mostly of precursors and not active enzymes worked best against cancer. Active pancreatic proteases present in the systemic circulation, as a start, appear susceptible to neutralization by a series of enzyme-blocking molecules called serpins present in blood. On the other hand, the proenzymes seem completely immune to such assault. Subsequently, at the cancer cell membrane—but not in normal tissues—the precursors quickly convert into their active conformation capable of attacking the malignant tissue directly and effectively. As they write in their abstract:

> We hypothesize that the provision of zymogens [proenzymes], rather than the enzymes, was of crucial importance to the clinical effectiveness in the human trials conducted by Beard and his co-workers. The precursor nature of the active enzymes may offer protection against numerous serpins present in the tissues and blood. Experimental evidence supports the

Gonzalez—History of Enzyme Treatment for Cancer

assertion that the conversion from proenzyme to enzyme occurs selectively on the surface of the tumor cells, but not on normal cells. We believe that this selectivity of activation is responsible for the antitumor/antimetastatic effect of proenzyme therapy and low toxicity to normal cells or tumor host. …These findings support the conclusion that proteolysis is the active mechanism of the proenzyme treatment.[35]

Though Novak and Trnka used only injectable enzymes in their studies, we believe the same rule applies to our orally ingested, largely unpurified, predominantly precursor product. We suspect a high percentage of the proenzymes do not undergo activation in their journey through the stomach and duodenum but remain in their inactive form to be absorbed as such. Then, after circulating unaffected by the various enzyme blockers in the blood, at the cancer cell membrane the precursors unleash a potent anticancer effect.

TWO CASES

In an article about our treatment approach appearing in the January/February 2007 issue of *Alternative Therapies,* I presented 6 unusual cases of patients diagnosed with poor prognosis or terminal cancer who had done well for prolonged periods on their nutritional regimen.[36] A lengthier version of the article posted on the *Alternative Therapies* Web site included 36 such case reports of our successfully treated patients.

Here we provide 2 more recent cases that were not included in the first article that we believe illustrate the continued efficacy of the enzyme-based therapy.

Patient 1: A Survivor of Stage IV Lung Cancer

Patient 1 is a 62-year-old man with a past medical history significant for elevated cholesterol, hypertension, and emphysema associated with a 35-year history of cigarette smoking, though he quit in 2001.

A computer expert by training, Patient 1 had been in good health before developing cancer. Despite a tough work schedule, he exercised regularly and followed-up with his annual physical exams at Kaiser. A routine chest X-ray in August 2008 showed "minimal insignificant thickening of pleura at both apices," which was discounted as being significant. But in August of 2009, Patient 1 first experienced persistent pain in his right-lower flank, the result, he thought, of pushing his exercise routine too hard.

The pain continued to worsen, and in October 2009 when Patient 1 first noticed bright red blood in his stool, he consulted with his primary care physician, who ordered CT scans of the abdomen and pelvis. The tests showed no abnormalities in the abdomen or pelvis but did reveal a right pleural effusion. A CT scan of the chest in mid-November 2009 indicated multiple pulmonary tumors as described in the radiology report:

... there are now evident multiple right pleural masses ranging in size from 1.5 × 4.0 cm down to 1.0 cm in the right lower chest with the largest pleural masses measuring 5.0 cm and 2.5 cm in the right pulmonary apex consistent with a Pancoast tumor. ... The 4.0 × 1.5 cm mass also destroys the adjacent right 7th rib in a permeative fashion consistent with metastatic disease.[36]

Two days later, an enhanced CT scan confirmed multiple lesions in the right lung, invasion of the seventh rib, and evidence of a left adrenal mass: "The central aspect of the left adrenal gland appears as a convex contour and this is suspicious for a mass that measures 1.0 cm."[36]

A fine needle aspirate of a right pleural-based lesion confirmed squamous cell carcinoma consistent with a lung primary. At that point, Patient 1's primary care physician suggested Percocet for his persistent pain, referred him to an oncologist, and arranged for a positron emission tomography (PET) scan, which in early December 2009 revealed evidence of significant disease:

> There is a hypermetabolic density in the right upper lung involving the pleura laterally and invading the chest wall at the level of the right second (2nd) rib (with possible bony involvement) with a max SUV [activity] of 14.6 measuring 2.9 × 2.3 cm. There as another nodular hypermetabolic mass involving the pleura in the right upper lung adjacent to the right fourth (4th) rib (max SUV 11.1 measuring 2.7 × 1.9 cm). There is a conglomerate of at least three (3) pleural-based hypermetabolic densities in the right lower lobe laterally invading the pleura and right lateral eighth (8th) rib. ... An additional similar pleural lesion is noted involving the anterolateral aspect of the right fifth (5th) rib ...
>
> There is mild focal increased activity in the distal esophagus with a max SUV of 3.7 and mild thickening of the mucosa. There is a right retrocrural node with a max SUV of 10.8 measuring 1.9 cm.[36]

The appointment with the oncologist went ahead as planned during the second week of December 2009. To evaluate the skeletal metastases, the physician suggested a bone scan which in mid-December 2009 indicated the following: "Findings consistent with osteoblastic metastasis within the right postero lateral eight (8th) rib, correlating to recent PET/CT findings. There is no evidence of osteoblastic metastatic disease elsewhere ..."[36]

With the workup completed, Patient 1 met again with his oncologist who explained that due to the extent of his metastatic disease surgery was not an option. Instead, he recommended aggressive chemotherapy with Taxol and carboplatin to begin as soon as possible, though according to Patient 1 he acknowledged the treatment at best would only be palliative, not curative, perhaps extending his life several months. With this information in hand and his disease considered incurable, Patient 1 decided against proceeding with conventional approaches. When asked, his oncologist admitted that without any treatment, he might live 6 months.

At that point, his doctors referred him for palliative care and to a staff acupuncturist for pain control. Patient 1 then went on a crash course of self-education about alternative approaches. He changed his diet radically, cut out junk food and refined carbohydrates, and began juicing and eating a largely plant-based 100% organic diet. He stopped the Zocor and Cozaar he had been taking for his high cholesterol and hypertension. Then in late December 2009, through a mutual friend, Patient 1 learned about my regimen, contacted our office, and because his attitude seemed so determined despite his situation we agreed to take him on as a patient.

I met with Patient 1 for the first time in mid-January 2010. He reported that his rapidly worsening fatigue had cut into his professional life, to the point he now could work no more than 4 hours a day before exhaustion would set in. In addition, he described severe right flank pain. He had not been taking the recommended analgesics because of side effects but was continuing with the acupuncture treatments, which he found somewhat helpful. I suggested that at least for now he continue the Percocet.

Thereafter, Patient 1 adjusted to the program well, though his pain at times could be unbearable even with Percocet. But gradually, Patient 1 began to improve. By April 2010, after only 2 months on treatment, he reported in a phone conversation that "the terrible bone pain" had completely resolved, so much so that he had been able to discontinue Percocet. He told me he felt great, and friends thought he looked "great." In fact he felt well enough to begin a vigorous exercise program at a local gym. A recent series of pulmonary function tests, according to Patient 1, were "perfect." And his blood pressure, off all medication, came in at 117/77.

I then saw Patient 1 and his wife in my office for his scheduled lengthy 6-month follow-up visit during the third week of July 2010. He looked, as my note from the session described, "wonderful," and he again reported feeling "great." He described his energy as "great" and stamina as "great," and he was sleeping well and could now work a full 8-hour day without difficulty. He reported that a recent cholesterol test at Kaiser was normal. I made some adjustments in his protocol at the time, and once back home, he continued with the same dedication to the therapy as before.

Thereafter, Patient 1 continued doing well. A year after his first visit with me, during the third week of January 2011, he developed severe right back pain in the area of his metastatic rib lesion. He faxed me a note reporting that the pain was quite severe and when we spoke by phone I did not like the sound of what he was telling me and insisted he needed a CT scan as soon as possible. That same day, CT studies of the chest and abdomen, his first since his initial workup in the fall of 2009, demonstrated pulmonary emboli in both lungs but no evidence of the multiple pleural-based tumors noted on the CT from November 10, 2009. A CT scan of the abdomen did reveal several small lesions in the liver, though the left adrenal mass seen on the enhanced CT scan from November 13, 2009 was not evident: "There are small hypodensities beneath the anterior liver capsule and the dome of the liver suggestive of early metastases. The spleen, gallbladder, pancreas, adrenal glands are normal …"[36]

With the diagnosis confirmed, Patient 1 was immediately started on Lovenox and Coumadin. The following day, ultrasound studies of his lower extremities revealed "an occlusive thrombus involving the right peroneal vein."[36]

With Patient 1 now stabilized, we had a long talk about the recent events. He said his doctors were dumbfounded that the lungs as well as the ribs showed no evidence of cancer whatsoever. Multiple radiologists had reviewed the scans, and there apparently was so much disbelief about the situation they had pulled out the original films to compare and re-evaluate. Indeed, despite their doubts, the multiple right lung tumors clearly seen in November 2009 were gone. And these had not been small tumors; the largest had measured 5 cm in widest diameter.

As for the small lesions now noted in the liver, the reports of the CT scan of the abdomen from late November 2009 and the PET scan from early December 2009 had not indicated any abnormalities in the liver. Patient 1 did not start his nutritional regimen until late January 2010, some 7 weeks after the PET scan. Because his disease was so aggressive, I suspected that during the time between the original CT and PET studies in November and early December 2009 and the time he started his therapy in late January 2010, his cancer would have continued to spread.

We also discussed the blood clots in some detail. As it turned out, I did not know the whole story when he had first called complaining of back pain. Just before he developed the backaches in the third week of January 2011, he had driven 12 hours nonstop to visit relatives in the midwest—a trip he had not discussed with me, assuming I would tell him not to do it. After several days with family, he then drove 12 hours back, again nonstop. I thought the clots easily could have developed during the long drives.

During the second week of February 2011, Patient 1's primary care physician arranged for an abdominal ultrasound to re-examine the liver lesions. The doctor's note to Patient 1 about results indicated the nodules seen on the January CT scan were gone: "Your ultrasound: No abnormal hepatic masses visualized."

I next saw him in my office in late July 2011, 18 months after his diagnosis, at which time he reported excellent energy, stamina, and concentration. His various pains remained completely resolved and he had resumed working 10- to 14-hour days without any drop in his energy. I advised him that he had to pace himself more reasonably and not try to conquer the world.

Today, in October 2014, nearly 5 years from his diagnosis, Patient 1 feels "great," with no evidence of his once widely metastatic disease.

Squamous cell carcinoma is one of the more aggressive of lung cancers, with fewer than 5% of those diagnosed at stage IV, as in the case of Patient 1, surviving 5 years. Considering the extent of his disease when initially diagnosed, Patient 1's current survival of nearly 5 years is unusual, particularly since he enjoys such excellent health. On his nutritional program his debilitating pain has completely resolved, his blood pressure and cholesterol have normalized without drugs, his energy is superb, and he continues his productive, creative life. Further, the regression of all his extensive lung and bone lesions after 1 year of treatment, and the subsequent resolution of his liver disease, certainly indicates a good response to therapy.

Patient 2: A Survivor of Burkitt's Lymphoma

Patient 2 is a 39-year-old woman with a diagnosis of Burkitt's lymphoma that failed to go into remission with chemotherapy, who has now survived 5.5 years on her nutritional regimen.

In terms of her family history, at least 7 of Patient 2's close relatives had been diagnosed with cancer, including her father with prostate cancer, a sister with cervical and skin cancer, a grandfather who died of leukemia, a grandmother who died from colon cancer, an uncle who died of lung cancer at a young age, a first cousin who died of colon cancer, and another first cousin with metastatic colon cancer.

Prior to developing lymphoma, Patient 2 had a distant history of allergies that developed when she was 10 years old and that her parents, with a long interest in nutrition, treated effectively with a whole foods organic diet and a variety of nutritional supplements. Thereafter, she did quite well, and throughout her 20s, she remained vigilant with her diet and health habits while also pursuing athletic and outdoor activities.

Patient 2 had been in her usual state of good health when in March 2008, she first experienced persistent low back pain associated with onset of drenching night sweats, diminished appetite, and weight loss of 10 pounds over a several-month period. During this time, she repeatedly consulted her family physician, who generally seemed unconcerned, though at one point he prescribed Valtrex when the patient herself suggested her symptoms might be due to shingles. However, the symptoms continued to worsen throughout late spring and early summer of 2008.

In early August 2008, over a period of several days, she developed a large mass "one-half the size of a football" in her lower back. At that point, Patient 2 was referred to a local oncologist in Washington State where she lived at the time. A CT scan in mid-August 2008 revealed an anterior mediastinal mass measuring 7.1 × 10.8 × 10.1 cm, compressing both the main pulmonary artery and aorta, and a mass adjacent to the spinal cord 5.7 × 7.4 × 7.4 cm invading the posterior chest wall and thought to be the cause of her back pain.

Two days later, a bone marrow biopsy was negative, but a CT-guided fine needle aspirate of the anterior mediastinal mass confirmed a B-cell lymphoma, positive for the CD20 antigen. Further molecular biology studies revealed a rearrangement of the c-Myc oncogene, which regulates cell division, via a translocation of chromosomes 8 and 14, or t(8:14). This finding helped confirm a diagnosis of Burkitt's lymphoma, a malignancy associated with Epstein-Barr infection, and rare in the United States though common in Africa.

By the time she was admitted to Providence St Peter's Hospital only several days after her biopsy, her clinical status was declining rapidly. A PET/CT scan at the time revealed the tumors had grown considerably in a week, the anterior mediastinal mass now measuring 15 cm, and the right paraspinal mass measuring 11 cm. In addition the PET revealed a new active 2.5 × 3.6 cm left ovarian mass and a 1.8-cm mass within the small bowel all consistent with metastatic lymphoma.

Patient 2's oncologist warned her that due to the extremely aggressive nature of her disease, she needed to begin chemotherapy immediately or she could be dead within 10 days. With no other immediate option, Patient 2 agreed to the treatment, the intensive McGrath protocol designed for patients diagnosed with Burkitt's lymphoma. The McGrath regimen consists of 2 courses, A and B, of multiagent chemotherapy given in sequence, the CODOX-M regimen A, and the IVAC regimen B. In this case, her physicians also opted to add on Rituxan, a monoclonal antibody targeting the CD20 antigen present on the membranes of certain lymphoma cells.

Only days later, Patient 2 began the McGrath A component with the drugs cyclophosphamide, doxorubicin, vincristine, methotrexate, and leucovorin rescue. Beginning on the first day of treatment, she also received Rituxan. In addition, she underwent intrathecal cytosine arabinoside (ara-C) to target any cancerous cells within the central nervous system.

After the first cycle of McGrath A, Patient 2's oncologist switched her to the McGrath regimen B (IVAC), including ifosfamide with mesna rescue, etoposide, and ara-C, which she completed in early November 2008. At that time, she also consulted with Dr Paul O'Donnell, a lymphoma expert at the Seattle Cancer Care Alliance (SCCA) at the Fred Hutchinson Cancer Research Center in Seattle to discuss treatment options. Dr O'Donnell recommended a stem-cell transplant as the only hope for long-term remission, suggesting immediate harvesting of her marrow stem cells to be kept in storage. However, he warned that for a transplant to be effective, she must enter into full remission first.

At that point, Patient 2 returned to St Peter's Hospital to complete another 2 cycles of chemotherapy. A PET scan in mid-November 2008 documented a significant response to treatment described in the radiology report:

Complete or near complete metabolic response in the anterior mediastinal mass with marked anatomic reduction in tumor size ...

Complete metabolic response in the right lower chest lesion with near anatomic resolution.

Complete metabolic response and anatomic resolution of mass in the left ovarian region and left lower quadrant bowel.

Patient 2 then returned to SCCA to complete the successful harvesting of her stem cells. Unfortunately, CT scan studies from mid-December 2008 showed that she was not yet in remission:

Within the anterior mediastinum adjacent to the ascending aorta and main pulmonary (sic) is a heterogeneously appearing mass with calcifications measuring 5.5 × 3.0 × 2.6 cm which has not significant changed compared to the November 11 examination

... The previously identified right paraspinal mass with atelectasis has decreased in size to 4 × 8 mm and now is only a small area of pleural or extrapleural thickening with a small amount of adjacent right lower lobe atelectasis.

Patient 2 eventually completed the full 6 cycles of McGrath A and B in early January 2009. But a restaging workup in late January 2009 again confirmed that Patient 2 had failed to enter remission, despite the aggressive treatment. CT scan studies of the chest, abdomen, and pelvis indicated that the anterior mediastinal mass, though somewhat reduced in size, had not completely regressed, nor had the pleural thickening and nodularity in the right lung base. A PET/CT performed the same day revealed increased activity in the mediastinum and pleura, consistent with residual malignancy:

Heterogeneously increased activity with max SUV of 4.5 is associated with 28 × 51 mm anterior mediastinal mass. ... There is increased metabolic activity with a max SUV of 3.6 associated with foci of right basal pleural nodularity and thickening. ...

Further, the main tumor had increased in size when compared with an outside PET performed in November 2008.

With that bad news, in early February, Patient 2 returned to SCCA for a meeting with an oncologist assigned to her case, who bluntly stated that because she had not achieved a full remission, her chances of a successful outcome with transplant were no more than 20%, with a significant possibility of death from the arduous treatment. According to Patient 2, this physician did not push chemotherapy because the odds of response were so poor. When her parents asked about Patient 2's prognosis, the oncologist admitted that without any further conventional treatment, she might live only 6 months.

The official oncology note from that session stated, "Therefore our interpretation is that the patient's disease is progressing under a debulking chemotherapy she received during the last few months." At that point, Patient 2 had already learned about our work from a friend and after discussing the situation with her parents decided to pursue our treatment.

When I first met with Patient 2 and her parents during the second week of February 2009, she appeared emaciated and was so weak she had to lie down on the couch in my office as I conducted my intake history. Her hair had fallen out from the chemotherapy, and she reported drenching night sweats requiring change of bed clothes 4 or 5 times nightly, chronic low grade fevers, headaches, and a persistent neuropathy, a side effect from her chemotherapy.

Despite her dire situation, Patient 2 proceeded with her nutritional therapy with great determination, great dedication, great enthusiasm, and, importantly, with full support of her parents. With all she had been through at her age, I marveled at her positive outlook and had nothing but admiration for her. She understood fully the severity of her situation but would do everything she could, she said, to "beat the odds." And within weeks of beginning the regimen, she reported a significant change in her health for the better. She felt strong enough she had begun riding a bicycle daily, telling me in a phone conversation she felt "like a million bucks."

CT scan studies performed March 31, 2009, after Patient 2 had completed only 6 weeks on her nutritional therapy, showed a significant reduction of approximately "50%," compared with the CT scan from mid-December 2008. The radiology report states:

> There has been decrease in the size of the anterior mediastinal mass which now measures 3.7 × 2 cm in transverse diameter, compared to 5.6 × 3 cm previously. There are more prominent calcifications due to treated lymphoma. There is somewhat less prominent, mild soft tissue fullness in the right paraspinal region at the T11 and T12 levels, without definite focal mass seen in this region.
> No significant mediastinal adenopathy or other mass are seen.

A chest X-ray ordered by her oncologist during the third week of June 2009 showed apparently near-total resolution of the mediastinal mass compared with an X-ray from early January 2009: "Impression/Decreased mild residual fullness of the left hilum and left AP window region./No acute cardiopulmonary process."

Subsequently, Patient 2 continued her program and continued doing well. All her previous serious symptoms—the anorexia, fatigue, night sweats, and weight loss—had resolved within months. In a phone conversation mid-January 2010, after she had completed nearly a year of her nutritional therapy, Patient 2 reported feeling "great." A PET/CT scan a month later, in February 2010, showed no residual or active lesions—she appeared to be in complete remission.

Subsequently, she has done very well. Although she had been warned before beginning her aggressive chemotherapy in August 2008 that the protocol would render her sterile, in March 2010 she called me to let me know she was pregnant. Throughout her pregnancy, she remained vigilant with her therapy, experienced virtually no symptoms, and in late December 2010 gave birth to a very healthy girl.

Today, 3.5 years later, both patient, now 39 years old and still on her nutritional regimen, and daughter, remain in excellent health.

I always learn much from my patients. From my first meeting with Patient 2, I was impressed with her positive manner, though she had been given a terminal prognosis, a terrible predicament for someone so young, and she was so weak during that session she couldn't sit in a chair. But her determination was evident, and her parents were both very supportive of her choosing our therapy. Patient 2 has repeatedly expressed her enormous gratitude for the therapy we make available as have her parents, who feel the treatment saved their daughter's life. Over the years, I have come to believe fully that the attitude of the patient, and the attitude of caregivers, are together the single most important determining factors between a successful outcome and failure. Patients at peace with their situation and grateful for each day, not filled with anxiety, doubt, and fear, always do the best. And supportive family and friends can make a huge difference in terms of the ultimate outcome.

REFERENCES

1. Porter W. Some practical suggestions on the treatment of diphtheria. *JAMA.*1886;7(17):454-455.
2. Beard J. The system of branchial sense organs and their associated ganglia in Ichthyopsida. *Quart J Microsc Soc.* November 1885;11:52-90.
3. Murray MJ, Lessey BA. Embryo implantation and tumor metastasis: Common pathways of invasion and angiogenesis. *Semin Reprod Endocrinol.* 1999;17(3):275-290.
4. Ferretti C, Bruni L, Dangles-Marie V, Pecking AP, Bellet D. Molecular circuits shared by placental and cancer cells, and their implications in the proliferative, invasive and migratory capacities of trophoblasts. *Hum Reprod Update.* 2007;13(2):121-141.
5. Stem cell. Wikipedia, the Free Encyclopedia. http://en.wikipedia.org/wiki/Stem_cell. Accessed May 6, 2008.
6. Wicha MS, Liu S, Dontu G. Cancer stem cells: An old idea—a paradigm shift. *Cancer Res.* 2006;66(4):1883-1890.
7. Wicha MS. Cancer stem cells and metastasis: lethal seeds. *Clin Cancer Res.* 2006;12(19):5606-5607.
8. Wicha MS. Breast cancer stem cells: The other side of the story. *Stem Cell Rev.* 2007;3(2):110-112.
9. Wicha MS. Cancer stem cell heterogeneity in hereditary breast cancer. *Breast Cancer Res.* 2008;10(2):105.
10. Terada T, Nakanuma Y. Expression of pancreatic enzymes (alpha-amylase, trypsinogen, and lipase) during human liver development and maturation. *Gastroenterology.* 1995;108(4):1236-1245.
11. Westrom BR, Ohlsson B, Karlsson BW. Development of porcine pancreatic hydrolases and their isoenzymes from the fetal period to adulthood. *Pancreas.* 1987;2(5):589-596.
12. Beard J. *The Enzyme Treatment of Cancer and Its Scientific Basis.* London: Chatto and Windus; 1911.
13. Beard J. The action of trypsin upon the living cells of Jensen's mouse-tumour. *Br Med J.* 1906;1(2297):140-141.
14. Rice CC. Treatment of cancer of the larynx by subcutaneous injection of pancreatic extract (trypsin). *Med Rec.* 1906;70:812-816.
15. Cleaves MA. Pancreatic ferments in the treatment of cancer and their role in prophylaxis. *Med Rec.* December 1906;70:918.
16. Campbell JT. Trypsin treatment of a case of malignant disease. *JAMA.* 1907;48(3):225-226.
17. Cutfield A. Trypsin treatment in malignant disease. *BMJ.* 1907;2(2435):525.

18. Roberts W. *Collected Contributions on Digestion and Diet*. 2nd ed. London: Smith, Elder & Co; 1897.

19. Beard J. Trypsin and amylopsin in cancer. *Med Rec.* June 1906;69:1020.

20. Levin E. Production of dried, defatted enzymatic material. *US Patent Office.* April 11, 1950 (No. 2,503,313):1-7.

21. Hald PT. Comparative researches on the tryptic strength of different trypsin preparations and on their action on the human body. *Lancet.* 1907;170(4394):1371-1375.

22. Wilhelm Conrad Röntgen--Biographical. Nobel Prize Web site. http://nobelprize.org/nobel_prizes/physics/laureates/1901/rontgen-bio.html. Accessed June 26, 2008.

23. Wilhelm Conrad Röntgen. Wikipedia, the Free Encyclopedia. http://en.wikipedia.org/wiki/Wilhelm_Rontgen. Accessed June 26, 2008.

24. Marie Curie. Wikipedia, the Free Encyclopedia. http://en.wikipedia.org/wiki/Marie_Curie. Accessed June 26, 2008.

25. Weinstein JW. Dr Beard's theory in the crucible of test: An experimental study of the trypsin treatment in cancer. *N Y State J Med.* August 1908;9:400-402.

26. Morse FL. Treatment of cancer with pancreatic extract. *Wkly Bull St Louis Med Soc.* March 1934;28:599-603.

27. Shively FL. *Multiple Proteolytic Enzyme Therapy of Cancer*. Dayton, OH: John-Watson Printing and Bookbinding Co; 1969.

28. Kelley WD. *One Answer to Cancer*. Los Angeles, CA: Cancer Book House; 1969.

29. Gonzalez NJ. *One Man Alone; An Investigation of Nutrition, Cancer, and William Donald Kelley*. New York, NY: New Spring Press; 2010.

30. Howell EH. *Food Enzymes for Health & Longevity*. Woodstock Valley, CT: Omangod Press; 1980.

31. Moskvichyov BV, Komarov EV, Ivanova GP. Study of trypsin thermodenaturation process. *Enzyme Microb Tech.* August 1986;8:498-502.

32. Legg EF, Spencer AM. Studies on the stability of pancreatic enzymes in duodenal fluid to storage temperature and pH. *Clin Chim Acta.* 1975;65(2):175-179.

33. Rothman S, Liebow C, Isenman L. Conservation of digestive enzymes. *Physiol. Rev.* 2002;82(1):1-18.

34. Liebow C, Rothman SS. Enteropancreatic circulation of digestive enzymes. *Science.* 1975;189(4201):472-474.

35. Novak JF, Trnka F. Proenzyme therapy of cancer. *Anticancer Res.* 2005;25(2A):1157-1177.

36. Gonzalez NJ, Isaacs LL. The Gonzalez therapy and cancer: A collection of case reports. *Altern Ther Health Med.* 2007;13(1):46-55.